A NEW GENERATION

Creating a Blended Family
through the
Power of Love

LILLY A. GWILLIAM

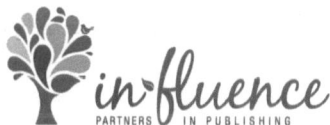

in-fluence
PARTNERS IN PUBLISHING

Published by Lilly A. Gwilliam
in partnership with Influence Publishing Inc., February 2023
ISBN: 978-1-7338997-2-7

Editing: Danielle Anderson
Proofreading: Lee Robinson
Typesetting and Cover Design: Tara Eymundson

DISCLAIMER

To the loves of my life:

My husband Gary, our children, and our grandchildren

*Your love has helped me be a more loving
wife, mother, and grandmother.*

Testimonials

"Lilly and Gary's story is a positively glowing example of what can happen when one takes a chance on love in midlife. . . . This love story shows us all how to live and what it means to be a family."

Elizabeth C. Saviano, nurse practitioner and health care attorney

❋

"Memoirs are special. And *A New Generation: Creating a Blended Family through the Power of Love* is particularly special because Lilly Gwilliam shares secrets from the heart and her courage to follow her intuition. It is an inside look into the mind of this passionate woman who examines, with honesty, her initial attraction to Gary Gwilliam, her trials and tribulations, her hopes for a wonderful future, and the courage to follow her intuition and overcome her fear of not taking action. It took great courage to write this book. All women can identify with the conflicting emotions expressed on these pages. . . . *A New Generation* is a keeper—definitely one you want on your bookshelf."

Jay W. Macintosh, a Californian attorney/actress/writer, retired and living in Paris, France

❋

"This sensitive, insightful, and concise memoir narrates not only of the challenges and rewards blending a complex family in midlife, but also of the author's tremendous drive to fulfill both her career and personal aspirations in the process. Lilly's story of determination, serendipity, and, above all, abiding love will be cherished by generations to come."

Paula Wagner, author of *Newcomers in an Ancient Land*, She Writes Press, 2019

"Lilly Gwilliam has brought us a story of personal wisdom and truth. In a stunningly descriptive chronicle of her life's journeys, her story draws a portraiture of love—love for her family, profession, and husband, Gary. Assuredly, you will be drawn in and stirred to reflect on your own life and those you love as well."

Maryanne Murphy, Esq.

"In her memoir *A New Generation: Creating a Blended Family through the Power of Love*, Lilly Gwilliam wrote: 'There is so much joy to share and so many ways to love in our family.' Obviously, these words uniquely relate to Lilly's blended family. However, I think this could also ring true for other families and/or relationships, whether blended or not. Lilly has captured the journey of today's blended family as she reveals her story to us. It's a story of trust, respect, and open communication, with joy and much LOVE mixed in. Her words have painted beautiful descriptions of the world she, her husband (Gary Gwilliam), and family have visited over the years. You'll be swept away to fascinating countries and lush island settings. It's like a mini travelogue! *A New Generation* made me think the essence of life is a voyage of discovery in more ways than one. . . .

"Lilly has created a must-read treasure while we sit in the front row observing 'the merging'—a.k.a. blending—of a lovely extended family!"

Lenore Kaler, artist/educator/marketing director/actress/realtor

"Lilly learns to blend the independence she developed as a single mother with her trust for Gary. . . . She tells the story of their maturing together and learning to deeply trust again. Although not everyone will have the kind of world travel adventures that they share, their example of including their children in their experiences is one that many could follow. As a result, Lilly is now able to enjoy this kind of loving relationship with her grandchildren that she experienced with her own grandfather."

Lynn T. Scott, Ph.D.

※○※

"Lilly's first memoir took us through the ups and downs of adolescence, parental relationships, and adult relationships. She established her career and emerged a single mother who was ready to take on the world. Now, in this memoir, her world is changed in a positive way when a prince charming disguised as a lawyer comes into her life. This romance blossoms like a rose, and one by one, the inner petals are revealed to us."

Ginny Mattson Crispell, retired English teacher

Table of Contents

Acknowledgments

I'd like to thank my loving husband, Gary Gwilliam, for standing by me during the time we have been together and while I wrote our story. You were always supportive of any idea I had—whether it was changing my career, traveling, or writing my memoirs—and you have sustained me as we have moved through our blended family story of love. I will never be able to adequately express how thankful I am to have you in my life.

To my children, Pat and Liz, thank you for your continued love and support, for sharing your lives with me, and for allowing me to be a part of your children's lives as well as your own throughout all these years. To Catherine, thank you for your openness to me as the new woman in your dad's life, for your support, and for your enthusiasm for my two memoirs. The same gratitude belongs to Lisa and Jen—while we faced some difficult changes when we first met, we have all come a long way in the past thirty years together. And to all of you, the arrival of each grandchild has not only enhanced our love among each other but also strengthened our family bonds. I love you all from the bottom of my heart.

I give another thanks to my middle-school dear friend, Lenore Kaler, for the support you gave me while I was writing my second memoir, and especially for helping me to try and find a title for my book while grieving the loss of your beloved husband, Robert Kaler. You have been my cheerleader since we were in the 4M Club back in the 1950s, and your enthusiasm for my writing these past ten years has been boundless.

A thank you also goes to my publisher, Julie Ann from Influence Publishing, and to Linda Joy Myers, my writing coach. Without your guidance and support, this book would not be in existence today. And thank you to Danielle Anderson, my editor, who has helped transform my story to be shared with all of you and helped me to continue writing my story when I thought I had nothing left to give. Thank you to Lee Robinson, my proofreader, who made sure my manuscript was ready for publication. I so appreciated Lee's professional expertise as to the correct grammatical reasons for the changes she suggested. And thank you to Anita Voth whose professional organization and marketing skills were a dream to work with and learn from for my book publication. I will be forever grateful for all of you coming into my life.

Introduction

In the late 1940s, when I was seven years old, I lived with my paternal grandparents for about a year while my mother and father worked to save money to buy a new house. My grandparents had immigrated to the States from Poland before starting their family, and I loved listening to their accents and smelling the scents of my grandmother's traditional cooking. She had two sisters who lived a block away, and they often would get together and share some "women talk." During these times, my grandfather—a tall, quiet, calm, and proud man who thought this gossip was nonsense—would come to me and say, "Agh! Come walk with me." We would walk together around the block, and he would share what happened at work that day. We ended our walks by sitting outside on the double-seated swing continuing our talks and just being. I felt so special and loved our time together. I remember seeing the love in their eyes as they looked at me through a glass window of their porch while I was playing teacher with my dolls, an experience that can never be taken away from me. In fact, it inspired me to become an adjunct faculty member of nursing many years later.

This experience shaped many of my beliefs around family. I saw how my grandparents supported my parents and how they treated me with such love and adoration. And I saw how hard my parents worked to provide for me and my brother Sonny during this time. As I approached adulthood and began picturing how I wanted my life to look, I knew that whatever else happened, family would be an important part of my life.

This foundation was further strengthened by the frequent contact with my aunts, uncles, and cousins during holidays and special occasions, especially my dad's side of the family. Both my mother and father shared the importance of family to my brothers and myself, and I am still close with all my cousins who live back east. I have also grown closer with relatives who live in other states over the ensuing years, even though visiting them is much more challenging. The values my parents instilled in me are further exemplified by my especially close relationship with my sister-in-law Carol Ann and nephews Jake and Tyler, who remain living in the home I grew up in after the sudden death of my younger brother, Guy.

During the early years of my life, my mother's side of the family was also very happy, and we shared many fun times together. However, as I detailed in my first memoir, *Generations of Motherhood: A Changing Story*, this side of the family slowly changed to the point where there was always some sort of drama or another, resulting in one or more family members not talking to one another over a period from several months to years. One sad result of this is that I was not informed of my grandmother's death until two years after she passed. I felt sad that I did not get to see her but was aware of this family dynamic and accepted it as it was. I also faced some challenges in my relationship with my mother, especially around my dream of pursuing a career in nursing. I still love this side of my family, but I decided a long time ago not to get involved in the drama, and to avoid passing on such dysfunction to my own children and grandchildren.

By the time I reached adulthood, I had a clear idea of what kind of a spouse and family I wanted to have. I knew family was of the utmost importance, and that it had to be similarly important to whomever I was with. When I first met my first husband, I was determined do things the "right" way: getting married and having kids even though it meant setting my dreams aside. It took many, many years for me to realize that I was a better mother, and a better person, when I took my own happiness into account. I had to learn that family was important, but I was important too, and I needed to find a way to balance both priorities in my life.

The story of finding that balance can be found in my first memoir. I had to redefine what family meant to me and what I wanted that to look like in my life. I also had to learn how to pursue my own happiness without relying on anyone else. It was a long and challenging journey, but I came out of it stronger and more settled into who I was. My children and I also had to adjust to this new dynamic in our relationship, and while there were some bumps along the way, we figured it out together.

In this book, my story comes full circle. Having learned to rely on myself, I was then thrown for a loop when I met my future husband, Gary Gwilliam, at the age of forty-eight. He showed me what a truly supportive relationship can look like by helping me pursue my dreams, even at his own expense. I no longer had to pick between family and a career; I could have both. Being with him also prompted me to redefine the meaning of family once more as we brought our five children together into one blended family.

My early life experiences with both sides of my family provided a strong foundation that gave me the strength to become the person I am today. They provided polar-opposite perspectives of what a family can be. I then combined this knowledge with my own experiences to build a foundation of love for my own children and grandchildren so they could feel confident going out and exploring the world, knowing that their family is behind them no matter what they choose to do in life. I was not the perfect mother, but I've done the best with the knowledge I've had at any given time, and the fact that we are all still so close speaks volumes to me.

These experiences have also given me the desire to create a record of the creation of my family for my children and grandchildren. I hope that this book will help them know Gary and my story and gain some of the perspective on family that I was so fortunate to receive from my own parents and grandparents. While we will all walk our own paths, I would like to think that they, and you, can take this story and use it as inspiration to find your own happiness, even if it looks different from what they or you would expect.

Life does not offer us the right person to spend the rest of our life with all packaged up with a neat little bow, nor does it give us all the answers as to where we will find love and joy. We need to be open to the signs of the universe around us and follow our intuition—only then can we find what we didn't even know we were looking for. I hope our story of love and family inspires you to take a risk and find happiness in ways you never expected.

ONE

The Phone Call

On a beautiful sunny fall day in November 1990, I drove from Glendale to San Diego to attend the California Trial Lawyers Association Convention. As a budding attorney looking to expand my knowledge, I had read up on this event and was excited to learn about the law and network with the interesting lawyers that I had become acquainted with from my time at the Los Angeles Trial Lawyers Association. I had recently taken the bar exam, and the results of the test were due to come out the Friday before Thanksgiving, which was two weeks away. As I drove, I envisioned myself becoming a member of the bar and practicing law within the next year. The view of the ocean as I entered La Jolla was endless, mirroring my feelings about the many possibilities that were opening to me with my combined degrees of nursing and law.

As I was driving, I reflected back on the significant turning points in my life. I was forty-eight years old with two grown children. My son, Patrick (also known as Pat), was twenty-six and was enrolled in the MBA graduate program at NYU in New York. My daughter, Elizabeth (also known as Liz), was twenty-three, had graduated from Chico State the past December, and was working at an insurance company in the Bay Area. I loved being a mother, and they were (and are) the most important people in the world to me.

Where had the time gone? It seemed like yesterday that I had divorced their dad, Ed, and obtained my Bachelor of Nursing, but it had already been sixteen years. Today I can see that our separation was not his fault; we married young, and we were both naive in many ways. I thought we wanted the same things when we first met, but as time passed, I realized that staying with him would mean giving up on my vision for my life. Unfortunately for him, that was not a sacrifice I was willing to make.

We separated in 1974, when the kids were eleven and seven, and I threw myself into my work. I went on to obtain my master's degree in psychiatric nursing in 1978, then worked at a large medical center in Chicago and joined the nursing faculty at Rush-Presbyterian-St. Luke's Medical Center. The time demands of my career created some difficulties in my home life, especially around Pat and Liz adjusting to their parents being separated. It was an emotional and painful time for all involved, and I'm glad that we eventually learned how to navigate this new dynamic and rebuild our relationships.

About two years after obtaining my master's degree, I realized that I needed a change. I was working with oncology patients at the time as well as teaching students, and while I loved both positions, I was getting burned out emotionally due to seeing my patients die over and over again. Rush-Presbyterian-St. Luke's was a high-achieving medical and nursing center, so it was common for my colleagues to move on and pursue their professional growth elsewhere after a certain amount of time. I knew it was time for me to do the same thing, but I was having trouble deciding what my next step would be.

After my divorce, I kept meeting men who were lawyers, and they kept encouraging me to apply to law school. I found this idea intriguing. At this time in our society, mental health patients were being supported by a group of lawyers and citizens who thought the mentally ill were being harmed by the mental health care system. They advocated that a mentally ill patient had the right to leave the hospital, and that a procedure would be established to assist them. As a psychiatric nurse, I knew there was another side of the law that was opposed to this approach. The fact that allowing patients to leave the hospital too soon meant they would end up returning shortly after being discharged because they were not finished with their treatment. This societal dilemma was of interest to me, so I decided to combine my psychiatric nurse background with the practice of law. I started law school in the fall of 1980, taking classes in the evening while working as a nurse coordinator at University of California, Los Angeles and sitting on the nursing school faculty for graduate students.

By the time I finished law school and began studying for the bar in 1990, I held two different nursing positions. I worked as a nursing supervisor at a mental health hospital in Long Beach every weekend from 7 a.m. to 7 p.m., and during the week I was a supervisor at another hospital from 3 p.m. to 11 p.m. This didn't leave much time for a social life, or to explore any other educational opportunities.

One day, I received notice that my weekend position was being eliminated, effective immediately. At first, I was in shock, but soon I felt tremendous relief, as if a weight had been lifted from deep within me. The first thing I did was to sign up for the California

Trial Lawyers Association Convention—the exact convention that I was now driving to. I was grateful to be able to take advantage of this unexpected opportunity: the educational programs would help me learn about the law, and the social networking would be beneficial to my future career.

Little did I know that this convention would impact more than just my job prospects.

During the opening luncheon, I found myself drawn to the handsome presenter with silver gray hair and eyes that reminded me of the Mediterranean Sea. He had been president of the California Trial Lawyers Association for the past year, and I could tell by the reception he was given—and by the award he was presented—that he was well-respected by the people in the room. I also learned from his acceptance speech that he had recently separated from his wife. For some reason, I couldn't help but feel proud of him, even though we had never met.

That night, a friend invited me to attend a candlelight meeting for lawyers who've had substance abuse issues—due to my background in psychiatric nursing, he thought I would enjoy sitting in on this meeting. Upon arriving, I was pleased to see Gary Gwilliam in attendance. He revealed that he had been sober for six years, and that he and his second wife had mutually agreed to get divorced after nineteen years of marriage because the two of them had grown apart. Gary had two teenage daughters, as well as a daughter from his first marriage. Now he was living alone for the first time in his life, and he was enjoying using his time to get to know himself. This resonated with many of my own experiences, and I felt I could relate to what he was going through.

As I listened to Gary, I admired the integrity that he showed in leaving his marriage. After listening to his story, I told him I was very impressed with the way he and his wife had handled their divorce and how they prepared their children for the change. He thanked me for my kind words. And at the end of the night, we parted ways, never to see each other again.

Or so I thought.

After I returned home, I couldn't get Gary Gwilliam out of my mind. Something kept prompting me to call him, even though the thought seemed absolutely crazy to me. First of all, I did not call men, especially one I'd only briefly met the night before. He was also recently separated, a recovering alcoholic, and lived five hundred miles away. Yet the thoughts persisted. After a few days and some prompting from my therapist, I finally worked up the courage to reach out and tell him—awkwardly, with a lot of stumbling—that I wanted to get to know him better. Thankfully, he felt the same way.

Two weeks later I found myself driving from Glendale to Oakland, still struggling to understand why I was traveling so far to meet a man I hardly knew. During the past two weeks we had talked on the phone a few times about ourselves, our families, and our career goals, but we were hardly more than strangers. Still, I felt a little thrill in my stomach at the thought of meeting him and pressed the accelerator harder.

In my excitement, I missed the exit and got lost, causing me to be about half an hour late. By the time I reached his building, I was flustered and anxious. I took the elevator up to the fifteenth floor and pushed the buzzer to his apartment. He greeted me looking as attractive as I remembered him to be, with his light blue eyes and silver hair that complimented his welcoming smile. I did my best to calm my nerves and embrace the strangeness of this day. I was unsure how this whole evening would unfold, but I was here. I might as well enjoy it.

He showed me around his two-bedroom apartment, with its stunning view of Lake Merritt reflecting the lights of downtown Oakland. A blue and tan sofa faced the floor-to-ceiling windows, which gave the room an open and warm feeling. As I sat down, I noticed a book about relationships on top of the glass coffee table: *The Journey of the Heart* by John Welwood. This gave me the impression he wanted to develop his ability to have a healthy relationship, which I considered a good sign. We chatted for a few minutes before heading out, and I began to relax and look forward to getting to know more about this man.

We went for dinner at a local restaurant, during which we talked about our children, the study of law, and our families. I felt unsure of myself at first; it had been many years since I had encountered a man who was actually interesting to me. I was used to dismissing the men who came on to me for being married, so I did not know how to confidently respond to a man who was available. But the more we talked, the more comfortable I became, especially once I saw how honest he was about his last two marriages and his role in how they ended.

When we finished eating, he invited me back to his apartment to continue our conversation. Once we arrived, he put on some Kitaro music and asked me to dance. I placed my head on his shoulder, enjoying the feeling of him next to me, and it felt like our bodies were the perfect fit. I pulled back and looked him in the eyes, and then he pulled me closer, and we kissed passionately. I felt as if I had known him much longer than one evening, or two weeks depending on how I was counting. At that point, time didn't matter. He stopped, looked at me, and said, "Lilly, I do not know if you will believe what I am about to say to you, but I love you." We sat on the sofa, and he held my hand. "I went to see a psychic last spring, and she told me my marriage was over and I would meet a woman who will be the surprise of my life. And I think that woman is you." I heard him, but I was unable to respond other than to continue to look at him with awe.

The view from Gary's apartment was beautiful, and the lights below were shining bright as we kissed once more. And despite my apprehension, I realized that I was excited to see how our story would unfold.

TWO

My Fantasy Weekend

As we pulled away from the kiss, Gary grinned. "Do you want to stay over here tonight?" he asked. "I have a pull-out sofa in the guest room. Or you can sleep in my new waterbed, which I think you would find much more comfortable."

I hadn't planned on staying the night as this was only our first date, but I'd had a few glasses of wine and was exhausted from the long drive. I'd also had a wonderful evening so far, and I felt comfortable with Gary. So, I decided that yes, I probably should stay. However, since I had not planned for this, I did not have a change of clothes or my toiletries with me. Gary lent me a shirt and a bathrobe to wear, and then he showed me the guest bathroom so I could have privacy while changing.

As I wrapped the large garments around me, I felt a little foolish. I could not believe this was happening. Everything I was doing in this moment was against my nature, against the way I had conducted myself for the last forty-eight years of my life. But Gary was sensitive to how I was feeling, and he helped me feel comfortable by laughing at our unexpected situation.

When I came out of the bathroom, he suggested we read the book I'd noticed when I first arrived. He sat next to me on the bed and read aloud until we were both tired, and then we fell asleep.

The next day, I awoke at my usual time of 6:30 a.m. I could not believe how well I slept and how relaxed I felt, especially since I was not used to seeing a handsome man's face on the pillow next to me. I smiled as I realized the previous night had not been a dream after all. Gary's bedroom window, which took up an entire wall, revealed an amazing view of Lake Merritt, with a sky full of clouds rolling by. The sound of the soft rain against the glass was intoxicating.

I got up and made my way to the small, cozy kitchen to find some coffee, as I usually did each morning at home. But as I searched through cabinets, I discovered that Gary didn't have any. I was still in Gary's shirt and bathrobe when he joined me in the room—apparently, he was an early riser too.

"How can anyone not have coffee in their kitchen?" I teased him. He looked so charming in his blue and white striped pajamas that I had to smile.

"I do have several choices of flavored tea," he offered.

"Oh no, not for me, tea makes me feel nauseous. Thank you anyway."

I had a cup of strawberry yogurt while Gary made himself some tea. Then we sat down at the kitchen table and looked at each other for a moment, as if we had found each other in the same dream. Finally, I broke the silence.

"Did you ever imagine we would be sitting here together this morning, with me wearing your shirt and robe? This is crazy."

Gary laughed, then tilted his head in a questioning manner. "What do you think of psychics?"

I wondered why he was asking me such a question. It seemed especially strange coming from a lawyer; I hadn't imagined a logical person like that would be open to such a thing. "I'd never thought much about them," I responded. "I know they exist, but I've never been to one."

"I know a terrific woman in Tiburon who does past life readings. Why don't I give her a call and see if she can see us today?"

This was becoming a very interesting day. I didn't know much about psychics, other than that I believed that they used their intuition to prey on vulnerable people. However, I was interested to know what Gary wanted to explore. And since last night's adventure had turned out so well, why not try another one? I agreed to join him, promising myself that I would do my best to keep an open mind. He called the psychic, who told him she was available, so off we went.

As we drove along in his light blue sports car, Gary explained that he'd started seeing this psychic a few months ago. Kay had a degree in hypnotherapy, and he found her to be very informative and helpful regarding his decision to end his marriage. This type of behavior was not typical of a left-brain attorney, so it caught my attention. As always, life is full of surprises.

Once we arrived, Gary and I walked hand in hand up to Kay's apartment, which overlooked San Francisco Bay. Kay was a slender woman in her mid-fifties. Her hair was pulled back with a clip, which enhanced her attractive face and warm blue eyes. She reached out her hand to welcome both of us into a living room decorated with oriental carpets and artfully arranged furniture. After offering us some tea, she directed us to sit on a three-cushion brown sofa before taking her place in a high-backed chair across from us.

Gary and I then took turns telling her about our meeting the night before and how amazed we were at the level of comfort we felt with each other. Gary asked if we might have any past lives together; he felt this might explain the connection we had.

Kay said, "Okay, let me see what I can find out for you." She closed her eyes and did some deep breathing; she seemed to be getting in touch with her spirit guides. After a few moments, she said, "You had a prior life in England, in the seventeen or eighteen hundreds. You lived on a large estate as brother and sister, and you ran the estate together along with your spouses." I smiled, thinking I could definitely see us running a business together at that time in history. I wondered what else she would find.

Kay then described a second life we'd shared where Gary was my father and we had a very good relationship. She added that this explains why I felt a warm sense of pride at the luncheon when Gary received the award. This past life idea resonated with me because I did feel an overwhelming sense of emotion for Gary at this ceremony, almost like a proud daughter would feel for her father, despite not knowing him yet.

Kay went on to say there was another life where I was a male priest and Gary a female parishioner. We'd had a torrid sexual relationship even though Gary was married to someone else at the time.

After the session with Kay, I still found the concept of past lives strange, but I was a little more open to the concept. It gave me some sense of why I felt like I had known Gary for a long time, and why Gary had said he loved me the night before. If nothing else, it was a fun idea to explore.

After we left Kay's apartment, we stopped for lunch and talked about our crazy weekend. We both started to laugh hysterically about the readings, to the point we had to leave the restaurant. The idea that we hardly knew each other and yet possibly had at least three past lives together was disarming and exciting at the same time. We found ourselves trying to grasp this new information and how it impacted the type of relationship that was possible for us. It was a lot to take in, and we couldn't help but get a little silly about it.

Eventually, Gary took my hand and said, "Look, I do not know whether you are my sister or daughter, male or female, but let's go back to my apartment." I nodded through the tears running down my face, unable to stop laughing.

By the time we came back to his apartment, the attraction had grown even stronger. So, we spent a wonderful day learning about each other. Gary was exciting to be with, and I enjoyed the feeling of his body next to mine. I had forgotten how beautiful and passionate I could feel with a man.

That evening, we decided to have dinner in and ordered Chinese food from a restaurant down the street. Gary's apartment was the ideal place for a quiet dinner, since the view allowed us to watch the magnificent sunset over the bay. As we ate, he said, "I called Steve after you first called me. I wanted to be sure that you were not his girlfriend. Steve is a nice guy, and I would never want to interfere with another friend's relationships."

I was surprised at his openness, but also happy that he shared this with me. "Gary," I told him, "you calling Steve reveals to me your integrity not only with Steve but within yourself and the people in your life. This is the same quality I saw the first time I met you at the candlelight meeting."

As we continued talking, Gary shared that he had started keeping a journal after he stopped drinking to help him get in touch with his emotions. The fact that he had been working on himself was most unusual in my experience—I had not met many men who were willing to look inside themselves. Gary was clearly an amazing man. I reached across the table to take his hand as he continued sharing his feelings with me.

"You know, yesterday, as I was waiting for you to come here, I wrote in my journal that this mysterious woman whom I hardly knew was driving five hundred miles to see me. I didn't know what the evening was going to bring, but I told myself that whatever happened, I was going to be totally honest with you. I was not very honest in my marriage, and now was the time to be totally open and honest in a relationship, no matter what the consequences."

As Gary spoke, I gained an even greater respect for him. I went to him and put my arms around him, feeling warm and loving. He held me tight and whispered he loved me, and we kissed.

After dinner, he told me he would be coming to Los Angeles the following weekend for a CTLA board meeting and would like to see me while he was in town. He also invited me to his law firm's Christmas party the weekend after. I eagerly said yes to both, happy that we were making plans to see each other again.

It was hard to leave Gary on Monday morning after our incredible weekend together. Everything was happening so fast. I felt like I was in a dream, like I was going to wake up and discover none of this was real. We held each other and kissed again before I got into my car to begin my long drive home. As I was driving down the I-5 toward Glendale, I thought about all that had occurred in the past forty-eight hours. Before leaving, I'd learned I'd failed the bar exam and was back to simply working to pay the bills. This news had left me feeling a little despondent and unsure of my future. Now a whole new landscape of possibilities had opened up to me, and I was invited to think more about what I wanted to do with my life.

After I arrived home, I kept smiling to myself as I thought about Gary. I was also pleased when he called that afternoon to check that I'd made it home safe and sound. I felt important to him, and I was beginning to think that the fantasy weekend might actually turn into something real.

THREE

The Mystery Woman

As I waited for our next visit to arrive, I decided to surprise Gary with a new hairstyle. I had changed my hair frequently over the years because I found it to be a creative and fun way to express myself, and because it symbolized whatever internal changes I was experiencing at that point in my life. This time, I decided to get a perm. I was now going to be traveling back and forth from Glendale to Oakland several times a month, and I knew a perm would be easier to maintain and style than my naturally wavy hair.

Finally, the weekend of the CTLA board meeting arrived. As I knocked on Gary's hotel room door, I couldn't help but feel a bit anxious; even though I liked my new hairstyle, I wondered if he would as well.

Gary flung the door open and grinned. "Who is this mystery woman here tonight?" His playful reaction made me feel beautiful. Then, as I entered the room, I noticed a bouquet of lilies in a vase on the coffee table. He smiled again and said, "I thought you would like these flowers, since they share your name."

I was so touched at his thoughtfulness. "This is the first time anyone ever bought me lilies," I replied. We put our arms around each other, and I sank into his embrace. I still couldn't believe how natural it felt to be in his arms, or how cherished I felt.

After simply enjoying each other's company for a while, we went to dinner at a Chinese restaurant and caught up on the past week over won tons and lemon chicken. We'd been talking on the phone every evening, but I loved that I could now see how he lit up as he looked at me. He sat back in his chair and looked at my hair with a twinkle in his eyes.

"I like it," he said. "So, what other surprises do you have for me? Will you be this enigma to me each time I see you?"

"No, seriously, this is it. I have to wait for this perm to grow out before I do anything else. I am happy you like it, though; it took me a while to get used to it."

Gary gave me an affectionate smile. "You will look beautiful no matter what hairstyle you wear."

We spent the weekend holding hands as we walked around the Santa Monica Pier. We talked about his past presidency at the CTLA, the practice of law, and the friends we had in common. For the first time in a very long time, I felt carefree and happy.

The following weekend, I flew to Oakland to attend his firm's Christmas party. This time, I knew that I would stay with Gary at his apartment, and I packed accordingly.

After I arrived, Gary told me something that I had not expected. He informed me that I'd be meeting two of his daughters at the party: Lisa, who was seventeen, and Jen, who was fifteen. He has another daughter, Catherine, from his first marriage, but she wouldn't be there that night. "They don't know about you," he explained, "but you might be able to find a way to subtly say hello and have a short conversation with them."

This reveal made me a bit nervous. I'd never been in a relationship where I needed to meet the man's teenaged children, so this was new and uncomfortable territory for me. Not to mention that Gary had just left a nineteen-year marriage a few months prior, so his two daughters were likely still adjusting to their parents being separated. I doubted they'd be expecting to meet their dad's new girlfriend right now.

In addition to this stress, I was also new to his law partners and friends. Not everyone would know who I was to Gary since his separation was such a recent event. However, he had told a couple of his partners about us, including Eric, the partner he opened the firm with in 1978. Gary said, "I told him the heavens had opened up and dropped an angel into my life." He wanted to introduce me to everyone and hoped I would feel okay meeting so many new people.

To be honest, I wasn't sure how I felt about it. I knew that everyone adored his wife, Liz, so it could be an awkward evening. Yet I was also excited to have this opportunity to learn more about this wonderful man.

Gary and I entered the party together, but he quickly disappeared into the room to greet his guests. Despite being left alone, I was surprisingly calm. After all, I had previously spent a lot of time attending functions with the Los Angeles Trial Lawyers Association, so I was used to being around lawyers. How bad could it be?

I noticed Gary's law partners standing together and went over to introduce myself. Among them was Eric, a good-looking, fit man in his early forties with gray hair at his temples. After I introduced myself, Eric said, "Oh you are the angel that dropped from heaven into Gary's life."

I smiled and said, "Yes, I guess you heard the story."

"Oh, yes! He is definitely smitten with you." I smiled again in response, not knowing what to say, though I felt he'd accepted me.

Also among the group was Jim, a friendly San Francisco-born Italian whom I'd met briefly at the convention in San Diego. He was very gracious to me and acknowledged me with a warm smile and a handshake. "It's good to see you again."

The other two partners, both named Steve, were friendly but reserved. They remained quiet, and I decided to move along and meet the other guests without bringing attention to myself.

There were about one hundred and fifty people at this very lavish buffet event. A large swan-shaped ice sculpture stood proudly in the center of the conference room table, surrounded by shrimp, carved sliced beef, cheese plates, meatballs, salads, chicken, and pasta. Cocktails and other drinks were available along with a fantastic array of desserts. The lighting was dim, and the sparkle of the lights on the Christmas tree and the energy of the guests combined to create a magical feeling in the room.

I got myself a glass of white wine and looked for friendly faces. I felt lost in this new crowd without Gary to show me around, and I was a bit confused. I had been alone at professional cocktail parties over the years as a single woman, but whenever I went to one on a date with a male friend, they stayed at my side and introduced me to people. While I knew Gary wasn't sure how to introduce me to everyone, I was surprised that he'd left me completely alone. I decided that I'd talk with him later about feeling abandoned by him.

In the meantime, I asked the people I met, "How are you connected to Gary and his firm?" I found this question helped break the ice because people were usually open to talking about themselves.

I soon became aware of both Lisa and Jen—Gary had shown me photos of them—but I didn't have the courage to start a conversation, no matter how small. What could I say to them without revealing who I was to their father? After a while, though, Lisa—a beautiful young woman with shoulder-length brown hair and blue eyes—walked toward me, and I decided this was the time to say hello.

"Hi," I said, "are you enjoying the party?" She responded with a smile. She introduced herself as Gary's daughter and told me she always enjoyed these Christmas parties. We chatted for a bit, during which she informed me she was a senior in high school.

"Do you plan on applying to colleges in the area?" I asked.

"Sarah Lawrence College is my first choice. I want to be a college professor, and I'm interested in the arts as my major." She seemed relaxed and comfortable with herself, but I wondered what she thought about the person asking her these questions.

Soon afterward, Jen came toward me as well. She was a tall, quiet, attractive young woman, and her brown eyes were warm and friendly. We also talked briefly, and she told me she was in high school.

I didn't want to bring any further attention to myself, so I soon excused myself and let them know how much I enjoyed talking to them. They never asked me who I was, and I was relieved to see that the evening went smoothly. It was an enjoyable and fun evening, and my concerns about trying to be comfortable faded away as the evening went on. Gary and I naturally came together at the end of the party, and we then hung out together until the night was over and drove back to his apartment together.

In the end, I didn't say anything to Gary about my feelings of abandonment. This was an unusual feeling for me to have, as well as a new situation for both of us, and I wanted to find out more about him before I said anything. Perhaps this is how events had gone when he attended them with Liz, and he didn't realize that he may need to approach things differently this time. I decided to take more time to learn about him and how he behaved and keep track of my feelings in the process. If I noticed this abandonment becoming a pattern, I'd address it then.

Gary talked with his daughters the following day, and he relayed to me that they'd inquired about the woman who was asking questions about their school interests. I guess I hadn't been as discreet as I thought. Gary told them we were dating shortly after, and they said they'd realized this was the reason I'd introduced myself. And since the separation from their mom was so recent, they also understood why he did not introduce me at the party. They didn't say much to Gary about how they felt about this new woman in his life; I hoped it wasn't too hard on them.

Gary and I were both quiet as he drove me to the airport a few days later. I was happy as I reflected back on all that had happened— meeting his partners and, more importantly, his two daughters—but I was sad to be leaving him for a week. "I'll miss you," I told him, breaking the silence.

"I'll miss you too," he responded. "I loved my time with you, though it was a very busy weekend. I hope I didn't overwhelm you with meeting so many new people."

"Yes, there was a lot going on, but I wouldn't have changed it. I loved being with you, and I'm looking forward to our next week together."

Gary looked at me with his loving smile, and I took his warm affection with me as I left on my flight. The love between us was undeniable. And yet . . .

As I sat on the plane, I examined my feelings for Gary and the way I was handling this relationship. Outside of him leaving me alone at the Christmas party, my time with him had been nothing short of wonderful—yet for some reason, I could feel myself putting up a wall. I loved him, but I was separating myself from those feelings, as if to protect myself from them. I had no reason to do this, no reason not to trust him, but it seemed to be an almost instinctual response to our deepening connection. I knew this was something I was going to have to explore and learn to move past if this relationship was to succeed.

Thankfully, I did not need to wait long for an answer. During our visits, Gary and I spent many hours talking about and reading spiritual books because we both gravitated to and enjoyed exploring our past and present lives together. Knowing this, Gary gave me a journal for my first Christmas gift since he found writing in one to be very useful for tracking his life and his growth as a person. Soon after, I wrote the following entry about our relationship and my insights about myself.

12-25-1990

It truly amazes me how the time goes by so quickly each year. As I approach the end of another year, another Christmas, I realize how hard endings are for me.

I like to pride myself with doing well with endings. But I have not done well with the ending of relationships, going back to my loss of my paternal grandfather when I was sixteen years of age.

However, now that I have changed this by meeting Gary and beginning a new and wonderful loving relationship, perhaps, through this journal, I can say goodbye to former losses and understand myself in a whole new and joyous way. Or, more importantly, accept my feelings of loss—sadness, heaviness— instead of denying these feelings and fighting the dark void I wish not to feel.

I found it interesting to note my eating behavior since leaving Gary on Christmas Eve. As soon as I returned to work, I started binging on sugars—candy, cookies, and yogurt. Ugh! I do not usually eat this stuff—I was not hungry and have never felt so fulfilled in my life as I have been in the past month with Gary. However, feelings of loss in leaving him and not being with him stirred some deep, unmet needs. God, I really feel awful. I do not want to continue to be so self-indulgent or destructive. I want to gain control and have faith in myself to handle these emotions, to allow myself to feel physically empty while emotionally fulfilled, which is how I feel with this love I have with Gary.

As I reread this entry, I can see that I felt vulnerable and wanted to dissociate from my feelings. Despite how happy I was, I did *not* want to acknowledge how much I was beginning to fall for this man. I still felt like I was in a dream, and like he was not real. Through this writing, I was getting in touch with my fear of getting close to a man the way I had been with my grandfather. I did not want to love anyone that much again, did not want to let them get close to me, because I did not want to feel that same hurt. Yet the beauty of this new love was the depth of it, something I had yearned for throughout my adult life, and I couldn't have this depth of love without giving and feeling. It was a real catch-22.

I wanted to trust and love Gary, and I was not afraid to do so on a spiritual level, yet I was subconsciously avoiding the physical pain of losing someone I really loved. My fear of loss was what I needed to work on if I wanted this relationship to grow.

We spent New Year's Eve with Gary's friend, Ed, and his long-term girlfriend, Pamela. I was looking forward to bringing in the new year with Gary, since my past New Year's had been spent either working or with friends.

I had arrived a few days prior, so we both got ready at Gary's apartment. I put on a long green and tan velvet dress that I loved, and Gary gave me an approving look when I walked out of his bedroom. "Wow, you look beautiful," he said. "I can't wait to show you off to Ed." He took my hand, and we drove into San Francisco to meet Ed and Pam at her condo.

Pam, an attractive woman with blond hair and blue eyes, met us at the door and welcomed us into the large living and dining room. Floor-to-ceiling glass sliding doors led out to a beautiful patio with a magnificent view of San Francisco, and the lights from the city reflected on the glass, creating a festive ambience along with the elegant white and gold Christmas decorations, lights, and candles.

Ed came toward us with his exuberant manner and again welcomed us to this lovely gathering. We sat next to each other on Pam's white sofa, beverages in hand—a glass of red wine for Pam and me and a glass of sparkling soda for Gary and Ed—and we got to know one another.

Pam's blue eyes sparkled, revealing her energetic personality. She talked with enthusiasm about her family's holiday plans, and she looked at Ed with love and adoration when she talked about how they met. I liked her immediately.

Ed, a handsome man with dark hair and a mustache, had been an instrumental part of Gary's life. A recovering alcoholic himself, he'd organized Gary's intervention for his drinking problem along with Liz Gwilliam. He was also very active in The Other Bar, an organization that supports lawyers who have a drinking problem.

Ed reminded Pam that I was the mystery woman he and Gary had met at the candlelight meeting in San Diego just six weeks prior, and Pam said she couldn't wait to hear the story. It was nice to no longer be this unknown woman who had entered Gary's world.

I enjoyed seeing Ed again, and the four of us had a fun and delightful evening bringing in 1991 at the Tonga Restaurant. We welcomed the new year with love and a true friendship that would last for years to come.

FOUR

Maui

On a sunny day in January, two months after we met, Gary and I flew to Maui from San Francisco. It was a dream come true; I had wanted to come to this beautiful island for a very long time. As we approached the end of our flight, the view from the plane amazed me. A few puffy clouds dotted the sky, and the water below was a clear, deep blue. The rich green mountains and grasses were reflected in the water below, presenting a unique beauty I'd never seen before. As we walked off the plane, a warm, moist breeze enveloped my body and spirit. I was in heaven. What a glorious feeling it was to have both life and love as we began ten full days together.

After we got the rental car, Gary steered us toward the condo we'd rented in Wailea. I sank into the seat as we drove, my senses pleasantly overwhelmed by the warm tropical breeze on my face, the rich colors of the grasses and bougainvillea bushes, and the beautiful scent of plumeria flowers. When we arrived, the warmth and desire between Gary and me created a rush to put away our luggage as soon as possible so we could relax in this beautiful paradise. The bedroom had an inviting queen-sized bed and a large window looking out over the spacious lawn and blue-green ocean. We fell into each other's arms and lost track of time.

Later, after we emerged from our room, we saw that the front door was still half open, and we hadn't taken the key out of the lock! We laughed so hard that my stomach hurt—we were acting like two teens at forty-eight and fifty-three. What a wonderful start to our vacation.

Gary and I walked hand in hand down the three-mile raised walkway along the Wailea beach, hoping to see whales, but it was too early in the season. That was okay with me; being able to spend time with Gary on this heavenly walk was more than enough. In one area, the waves were splashing up on the path, and we walked through it knowing we would get soaked. We yelled out in glee at this jolt of cold water and then laughed at each other, both dripping wet. The trip was becoming quite an adventure in unexpected ways.

Everywhere we walked, the view was magnificent. There were several other Hawaiian islands visible in the distance, and children were squealing with laughter as they ran along the beach. Dog owners tossed sticks into the turquoise water, and their dogs ran excitedly to fetch them. We walked barefoot, enjoying the feeling of the green grass and soft sand beneath our feet.

Some of our trip was planned out—we knew we wanted to stay in Maui for one week, and we planned to attend a trial lawyer conference happening in the area—but we also allowed for some free time to explore the island. On our third day, Gary had a suggestion. "I think you should experience the drive to Hana," he said. "My college fraternity brother, Kris Kristofferson, lives there with his family. Kris is out of town right now, and I hope we can see him another time, but I think you'll love this part of Maui—it's very tropical compared to Wailea. We could spend the day driving there and exploring the other side of the island." I could see that Gary was eager to show me all around the island, so I agreed to stay overnight in Hana.

While we didn't get to meet Kris on this trip, I am grateful that we did eventually get to meet him and his wife, Lisa, a year later. It was exciting to see Kris drive up in his truck to meet us at the Hana airport, and I quickly learned that he was very down to earth and funny. He and Gary talked about some of their fraternity brothers and what was happening in their lives. Lisa had also gone to law school, so she and I had a lot in common between being a mother, wife, and law graduate. We had a wonderful day together and have kept in touch throughout the years.

The brochure for Hana stated that it was located at the eastern end of Maui and is one of the most isolated communities in the state. To get there, you have to take the Hana Highway, which is a long, winding, fifty-two-mile drive along Maui's northern shore. It was described as one of Hawaii's most scenic but toughest drives. I tend to get car sick and was unsure about how I would react to the winding roads, but I didn't want to dampen his enthusiasm. So, we got some anti-nausea medication and set off.

The drive was definitely a queasy one for me, even though Gary drove slowly around the curves. I had to take deep breaths with the window open to keep the nausea at bay, and we stopped for a break to help get my bearings. But in the end, we made it through.

Upon our arrival, we discovered that Hana was a quaint little town surrounded by lush, tropical trees with three restaurants and a few small stores to shop in. Gary slowed the car right down as we approached the address for our rental, and we finally came to a long driveway surrounded by bushes, with the house well off the main road. At the end of the driveway, we discovered a small, weathered house that looked like it could use a serious face lift. Both of us stared at the place, unsure what to do next.

Gary spoke up first. "This is not what I expected. It looks very different from the pictures I saw online."

"Do you think this is the right place?" I asked, dismayed.

He checked the address again. "I think this is it, and I think we're stuck with it. I haven't been to Hana in years, and there were no other places available."

Despite our hesitations, we decided to head in. I felt distinctly uncomfortable, but I was willing to see if it might work. After all, it was getting late, and it would be too difficult to drive back along those curvy roads in the dark.

Gary held the door open, and I walked into a dreary room that was so humid I could hardly breathe. The living room held a funky green plaid sofa and chair, and the tiny bedroom had a small window that was blocked by overgrown bushes.

I took a deep breath, then turned to Gary. "So, what do you think?" I was doing my best to stay calm, but in my head I thought, *Are we really going to stay here?*

Gary looked at me with concern. "Well, it's not quite what I expected, but it might be okay for one night, if it's okay with you."

Pushing my concerns aside, I assured him we could stay. I didn't want him to feel badly about his choice, and really, how bad could it be?

After we settled in, we strolled down the road to look at the beach, then sat on some rocks along the water's edge to eat our take-out dinner. We enjoyed another amazing view of the ocean, and the sound of the waves crashing against the shore lifted my spirits, though I still dreaded going back to the house.

We spent the rest of the evening in the living room, relaxing and attempting to read as the barely functioning ceiling fans stirred the humid air around us. The lighting was so dim that reading was nearly impossible, but there *was* enough light for me to notice several small creatures on the wall.

I freaked out. "What is that?" I screamed as I sat motionless, afraid that whatever I was seeing would crawl on me.

Gary checked what I was looking at, then laughed. "Oh, they're geckos, and they are good to have around because they eat all the bugs. They won't hurt you."

"I don't care. I've never seen them before, and I don't like them." Unfortunately, despite my protestations, the geckos were here to stay. I watched them from the sofa with zoom-like focus for the next while, on the alert for any movement in my direction. I was never a bug person, and to me, these fell squarely within that category. Gary was very supportive of my concerns, though, and helped me remember that I am bigger than these little creatures. I still didn't like them, but I learned to tolerate their presence.

I was beginning to welcome sleep after the long day. As I passed the tiny kitchen on my way to the bathroom, I turned on the kitchen light and noticed little brown things scurrying under the refrigerator.

"Gary, please come here!"

"Yes! We have cockroaches," he said, completely unphased by their presence. He also didn't like them being there, but he tolerated it better than I did.

Gary tried to use logic and reasoning to help me overcome my fear of these creatures. He told me that they wouldn't hurt me, and that we just needed to get some rest and then we could leave early in the morning. I doubted that I would sleep, but I snuggled close to him and tried to relax. Morning couldn't come fast enough. Yet another unexpected adventure, though I wasn't sure I liked this one as much as the rest.

※

Then next morning, Gary said, "How would you like to drive to Kapalua on the other side of Maui? We can meet up with some lawyer friends of mine who are attending the American Trial Lawyer Association seminar." I happily agreed. Having survived the night, I was ready to leave and have more adventures—hopefully with less bugs. I was also eager to see another part of this beautiful island and meet Gary's friends.

On our drive to Kapalua, I enjoyed seeing the casual lifestyle of the Hawaiian people and the multi-colored muumuu dresses worn by the women. The pace was slow compared to the hustle and bustle of the Bay Area; the people we passed seemed relaxed and happy and were quick to smile and wave as we passed by. As we drove from one side of the island to the other, clouds hovered over the mountains with threats of rain, then retreated to allow the sun to shine through. It was magical.

At one point on our drive, Gary said, "Let's go shopping for some fun clothes and souvenirs. There are some very nice shopping areas ahead, perhaps it would be fun to take a break and walk around for a while." He grinned at the thought, but I didn't know how to respond—I had little money to spend.

After a short pause, I answered, "Hey, I'm fine, I don't need anything. If you want to shop for your daughters, that would be all right. I'm happy to help you pick out something special for them."

"No, I want to buy something for you."

Once again, I didn't know how to respond. A man hadn't bought something for me for a long time. "Gary, I don't need anything. I'm enjoying this trip so much."

"Let's go and look at what's available," he insisted. "If you don't like anything, that's fine." I agreed to look, but I felt awkward and uncomfortable. Men didn't usually shop with me, and I didn't really want him to buy something for me when I couldn't afford to buy anything myself.

We found a store to stop at, and Gary kept urging me to look at various dresses. I finally decided to try on a two-piece green and beige floral Hawaiian dress with a skirt that hit just above the knee. He wanted me to show him how it looked on me, and as I stepped out of the fitting room, I felt so foolish. What if he said he didn't like it? I would feel so ridiculous! I was uncomfortable being looked at and felt exposed.

"Okay, here I am, but I'm not sure about the short skirt. What do you think?" My face was flushed, and my voice was meek.

"I love it!" he said, grinning and giving a thumbs up in approval.

"Don't you think it's too short?" The skirt was formfitting, sexy, and so unlike my usual outfit of pants and a jacket. I was way out of my comfort zone, but Gary assured me that it was a good length.

Throughout this process, I was surprised about how many mixed emotions I had to overcome after sixteen years of living on my own. It was amazing to me that I could get to be a forty-eight-year-old woman—someone who'd experienced marriage, motherhood, and divorce, who'd become a professional nurse and was now pursuing a career as a lawyer—and still feel like an adolescent around a man I had feelings for. I wasn't sure how to act around him. Wanting to enjoy this time with him, I did my best to push away these feelings and embrace this new way of being with someone.

As we were checking out, Gary suggested that I wear my new outfit to meet his friends that night at the Hyatt hotel. I told him I wasn't comfortable wearing it around people I didn't know, and Gary smiled again. "Oh no, you will be fine to wear it since Maui is so casual." I thought on this as we drove to the hotel, and by the time we got there, I became comfortable with the idea. I liked how the green pattern of the dress accentuated my green eyes, and it was fun to explore a way of dressing that was more casual than my more formal professional look.

The gathering at the Hyatt was surprisingly relaxed, and the people Gary introduced me to were very gracious and welcoming. Most of them were surprised to meet me because they didn't know Gary had separated from Liz, but it was never awkward since I had nothing to do with their relationship ending. I was delighted to see some familiar faces from the Los Angeles Trial Lawyers Association, and I enjoyed spending the evening connecting with friends, both old and new—and spending time with Gary, of course.

The morning of our flight home, we finished packing at our lovely condo by the beach. Gary took me in his arms, and I said, "I never imagined this trip with you would be so wonderful. I had a fabulous time, and I loved all our time together." We held our embrace, feeling so much closer after ten days of being together.

I was completely unprepared for what came next. "I was thinking the same thing," Gary replied, "and I wondered . . . would you consider living in Oakland? With me?"

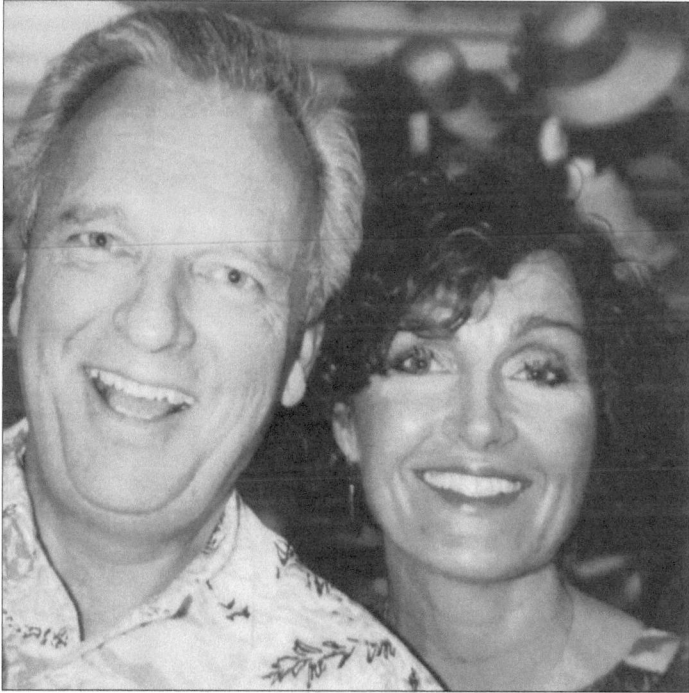

Lilly and Gary in Maui, 1991

FIVE

Connections

On March 1, 1991—four months after meeting Gary—I was excited to be moving my belongings from Glendale, where I'd been living for about two years, to Oakland so we could live together. It was a surprising turn of events, especially since our whole relationship had unfolded so quickly, but we felt we were ready.

One Saturday evening, shortly after I first moved in, I was sitting on the sofa writing in my journal while Gary was sitting in a lounge chair across from me reading *The Journey of the Heart*. It was one of the few quiet evenings we'd had together, and I was thoroughly enjoying it. This was the kind of life I'd always wanted but didn't know was possible.

However, something was niggling in the back of my mind. Throughout the time we had been seeing each other, my throat would become constricted and painful every time I left Gary to go back to Los Angeles. I also found it very difficult to be apart from him for any length of time. I felt an overwhelming love for him, and

I feared the possibility of losing him. We had assumed that I was experiencing this because we enjoyed being together, so now that we were living together it shouldn't happen very often. But what if there was more going on? I was curious. And now that we were living together, we weren't trying to cram as much as we could into our limited visits and had more time to explore something like this.

Finally, I got Gary's attention and asked, "What do you think about seeing Kay for a reading to explore why my throat tightens up every time we part?" Where her previous past life reading had helped explain the connection Gary and I had, I wondered if she may be able to help us in this matter as well.

"Great idea," he responded. "Let's see if she's willing to come here, to our place."

A few days later, Kay came over for a session. She expressed pleasure at seeing us in Gary's apartment and hearing the story of how our relationship had progressed.

Kay started this session by sitting quietly across the room from us, eyes closed, hands resting on her knees, palms held open. After a few minutes of silence, she said, "I see you and Gary in your early twenties, living in a place perhaps in Sicily. You were engaged to be married and were horseback riding when lynch men came upon you from behind and, Lilly, slit your throat before literally dragging Gary away, leaving you to die."

We sat there in silence, each of us trying to take in what she said. It was such a violent image. Gary reached over and gave my hand a squeeze to comfort me and express his love for me.

After the reading, I felt a lot better about what I had been experiencing. Knowing the possible story behind my symptoms seemed to release my fear of losing Gary, and the constriction in my throat

disappeared. I also noticed that some of that wall I had built to protect myself had come down, and I was able to express my love and
thoughts toward Gary much more freely.

After moving in with Gary, I needed to find a job while also making
time to study for retaking the bar exam in July. As a people-pleaser, I
knew the latter would be difficult for me. For the past sixteen years,
I hadn't needed to consult anyone about the decisions I made or
how I spent my time. Now I was in this new relationship, and I was
struggling with my fear of being vulnerable. I was going to have to
set limits so I would have time to study, and I had to trust that this
plan to retake the bar exam would work for both of us. I could also
see that the only way to move forward was through open and honest
communication.

I had been reading *Personal Power through Awareness* by Sanya
Roman, which reinforces our power to act as our higher selves. I
interpreted this approach to life as living authentically and thinking
positively. I was struggling to stay positive, though, because I was
worried that I'd made this big leap without knowing Gary very well.
I'd not only become emotionally invested in this relationship, but I'd
also given up my job and life in Los Angeles to be with him. What
if it didn't work out?

I was dependent on Gary in these early weeks, and I didn't like
it. I tried not to show my fears—I wanted to work through them by
myself. And truthfully, part of me was concerned he might become

interested in another woman if our relationship was less than perfect, like I had seen happen to several good friends of mine over the years.

Despite these fears and misgivings, our relationship only seemed to strengthen with time. Gary and I wrote love notes to one another every day and left them in different places for the other person to find. Every evening we walked around Lake Merritt and watched the herons swoop in to catch small fish for their dinner. There were geese everywhere, and the sounds of these birds were a reminder that we were a part of an animal kingdom that existed all around us. As we took these delightful walks, we would dream about the trips we would like to take together. Gary and I discussed the places we would love to see—Africa, Poland, England, and Alaska were at the top of the list.

One thing that was clear was that Gary wanted to live in Oakland for the foreseeable future. Gary still cared for Liz and his daughters as well as his beloved dog, Sam. They all lived in the Oakland hills, not far from his apartment, and he told me he wanted to stay close so he could be available to them. I very much respected him for this—he'd left his marriage in a loving way and remained the caring man I knew him to be. I could still remember how hard it was for Ed to leave the children and move out from the house he loved after our separation.

Staying in the Bay Area worked for me as my own children, Pat and Liz, planned on returning to San Francisco after college. Their father, Ed, also lived in the Bay Area, so the kids could now easily see both of us in one trip. Liz was especially happy with my move as she lived in Pleasanton, California, just a forty-minute drive away. Neither of them had met Gary yet—our visits hadn't included enough time to see Liz, and Pat was attending graduate school in

New York—but they knew of our relationship. Liz and I talked often, and she was happy that Gary and I seemed to be doing well.

I also hadn't had a chance to introduce Gary to many of my friends yet; due to the nature of our relationship and his busy legal practice, my life was quite consumed with his world at this time. He did get to meet my friend Suzanne, who I attended nursing school with back in 1971. She and I also got divorced at the same time. Her second husband, Sherwin, had also been previously married and had children from his first marriage, while Suzanne had two children of her own. This gave us all a lot in common, making for easy conversation. We had a delightful evening with them that included many laughs, and I was glad to expand Gary and my relationship in this way.

A month after I moved in, I met Gary's half sister, Patsy. She had not seen Gary since their mom died several years prior, and after hearing about us moving in together, she wanted to meet me and to see where her brother was living since separating from Liz. We met at Gary's apartment, and she was so excited to be there with him and to meet me. I was happy to meet her as well.

Gary had shared stories with me about his sister prior to our meeting. Patsy was six years younger than Gary and her father, Wayne—Gary's stepfather—had been very critical of her since she was a young girl. This was naturally very hard on Patsy, and she grew up with a low self-esteem as a result. Gary was shielded from Wayne's influence since he was beloved by his maternal family. While he went on to become a successful lawyer, Patsy became a teenage mother and did not attend college. Gary admitted to me that he too had not always been nice to his sister, even though she adored and looked up to her older brother. I looked forward to meeting her and knew that Gary felt it was time for him to make an effort to be there for her since their mother had passed away.

Patsy lived in Ogden, Utah. She had long, dark hair and an infectious laugh, and her upbeat attitude made her easy to be around. Upon meeting me, she said, "You probably have heard terrible stories about me. I'm the sister quite unlike Gary. I'm the black sheep of the family!"

I laughed at her openness. "I am so happy to meet the infamous Patsy."

I really liked Patsy right from the start. She was open and honest, and I could relate to her instantly. She was funny and didn't have a filter, so you never knew what she might say next. Her voice was rough, raspy, and loud, but her eyes twinkled with a mischievousness that was charming. It was as if she embraced being the "bad" sister.

The three of us had a fun weekend together just hanging out and going out to eat. Patsy worked sporadically, which meant money was an issue for her, so Gary covered her meals since she was our guest. As a result, she was like a kid in a candy store every time we took her out. She would pore over the menu, delighted to know she could order whatever she wanted without having to worry about the cost.

This visit gave me the opportunity to learn a lot about Gary's childhood. I loved hearing Patsy's perspective on life with their mother and Gary's stepfather. I was also saddened to learn that Patsy had lived a hard life, getting involved in drugs as a young woman, and that her daughter seemed to be traveling a similar path. During one dinner, Patsy said, "My daughter is a sweet young woman, but like me, she's a high school graduate with no goals for her future. She is just drifting now and hangs out with a drug group. I hardly ever see her."

After Patsy returned home, Gary and I reflected on the time we had spent with her, and he was able to provide a bit more context around the struggles she and her daughter faced. He said they both were kind, caring young women, but they lacked self-esteem and had a hard time believing they were worthy of love. Regardless, I could tell that it was important for Gary to have Patsy as part of his life. And now that I'd met her, I knew I'd always support their relationship.

Meeting Gary's sister made me reflect on my relationship with my two brothers: Sonny, who is fifteen months younger than me, and Guy, who is eighteen years younger. They both were hard-working men with careers in the construction business in New York, which meant I did not see them very often. We did not have much in common, but I did keep in touch with Guy, often catching up with him over the phone, since he had never left home and was still living with my mother after my father died in 1982. My brothers were both married and had families: Sonny had a daughter, Angela, while Guy had two boys, Jake and Tyler, with his wife, Carol Ann. I would go back to New York to visit them about once a year.

While I was becoming closer with Gary's family, I started to feel a barrier forming between myself and Gary's friends and colleagues. People had initially been very welcoming of me when I entered Gary's life, but it was now becoming clear that questions and rumors were circling. Gary met me only six weeks after his marriage ended, and four months later I was living with him. Everyone was quite surprised by this, including his wife, Liz. I sensed that people assumed Gary and I had known each other before he and Liz separated, and that they might have thought I was the reason he left her. It was hard to navigate all these layers of Gary's life, and it was a difficult time for everyone involved—myself, Gary, Liz, and their kids.

A year after we started seeing each other, Gary and I were having dinner with a close lawyer friend of his when his wife quietly leaned toward me and asked, "Did you know Gary before he separated from Liz?" Her honesty and curiosity reinforced my belief that almost everyone around us was asking this question. And it was hurtful to know people thought this of me, because my ethics would never allow me to play a role in breaking up another couple's marriage.

Some relief from this turmoil came after I wrote my first memoir, *Generations of Motherhood: A Changing Story*. After it went to print, I received an email from one of Liz's family members. He'd read my memoir, and he wanted me to know he was happy to see I'd had nothing to do with the breakup of her and Gary's marriage. Hearing those words meant everything to me. In that moment, I learned about the power of speaking my truth and having it acknowledged.

Despite my underlying insecurities in that first year with Gary, I had fun with him and loved him with all my heart. We enjoyed sharing conversations about the legal world and spending time with our mutual friends. And as our relationship strengthened and blossomed, our trust in each other strengthened as well.

One of the first professional meetings we attended together was a CTLA board meeting in Silverado, just over two months after we moved in together. As we arrived at the hotel, Gary said, "How would you like to drive my convertible around wine country while I'm in the meeting?"

Surprised, I said, "Are you kidding me? Are you really going to let me drive your precious car?" I was so thankful and felt empowered by Gary trusting me to do this—he had never let any other woman drive it before.

Gary got out of the car and motioned for me to sit in his seat. He showed me how to shift the gears, and I was happy that my prior experience with manual driving came back so naturally. We hugged and agreed to see each other at the group dinner that evening, and then I drove off on my own. I loved that he trusted me enough to let me spend the day exploring wine country in his beloved Mercedes.

A few weeks later we went to Scottsdale, Arizona, to meet with Gary's stepdad, Wayne, as well as some other family members. As we drove from our hotel to meet his family, Gary filled me in on a bit of their history. He told me that Wayne originally lived next door to their family and married Gary's mom when he was two years old. Wayne did not care to be a father and was quite the ladies' man, and he was unfaithful for a few years of their marriage. He became a better husband to Gary's mother in her later years, after she became ill with a heart problem, and they stayed together until she died in 1988.

Gary then explained that Wayne was not a great father figure. "I never liked Wayne, and he never wanted children. Patsy, my half sister, was born six years later, and Wayne was a terrible father to her. He was never there for her or me, emotionally or physically, and he would ridicule us. Wayne made fun of her for being overweight, and when I thought I'd like to play the trumpet like he did, he laughed and made fun of me. I never tried to play the trumpet again."

I said, "He sounds like a character. How do you feel about seeing him now?"

"I am okay with him since I do not see him very much," Gary replied, "and I want to stay in contact with him because Patsy and her daughter live nearby, along with my two aunts whom I was very close with growing up." These relatives all lived in Ogden, Utah, and would spend a few months at Wayne's trailer park every year.

We arrived at the trailer park, which was a small, tidy retirement community nestled in the dry Arizona landscape. It was early spring, so we met the family outside of Wayne's trailer under the roof of a carport.

Wayne was a small-built man in his eighties with a full head of thick gray hair. His tan, wrinkled face was weathered from the sun, but I could see he had been good-looking as a young man. And from the moment I met him, it was clear that he was quite the character; he greeted Gary by giving him a wink and a thumbs up.

Gary also introduced me to his uncle Vince and his wife Sue, his aunt Rose, and his uncle Ralph. The weather was perfect for sitting around the table and enjoying the sunshine, snacks, and drinks as everyone shared stories from Gary's childhood. I laughed as I heard about all their family dynamics, including a crazy grandmother who played all the siblings off one another. This made me feel connected to everyone, since my maternal grandmother acted in much the same way.

For example, Sue shared how Gary's maternal grandmother did not like Vince's first wife; the two women apparently never got along. When the divorce happened, Vince's wife brought a lawsuit against her former mother-in-law for alienation of affection. She claimed that the marriage had failed due to the hostile behavior from Vince's mother, and that she could never do anything right in her mother-in-law's eyes. She claimed this ongoing hostility had affected her relationship with Vince and ultimately lead to their divorce. The court ruled in favor of the ex-wife, and she was awarded a sum of money.

There was a similar story on my maternal grandmother's side of the family. My grandmother had seven children and, as she became older, would play one child against another. When my grandmother was living with my mom, my grandmother called my aunt, who lived one town away, and said my mother was not being good to her. The result was my aunt came to my mother's house and literally took my grandmother away to live with her instead. There was no communication or explanation about why my grandmother was moving, and my aunt wouldn't talk to my mother for several years after that, to the point that I didn't know my grandmother died until two years after it happened. As much as it was nice to feel this shared connection with Gary's family, I was determined that neither Gary nor I would continue this family dysfunction.

Overall, the time we spent with Gary's family was delightful. I enjoyed meeting Gary's family and connecting with them all, and I appreciated having this chance to see Gary in a new light. I also enjoyed learning more about what his childhood was like. Every new thing we learned about each other brought us closer together and strengthened our connection, and I'm glad for every opportunity we've had to grow together.

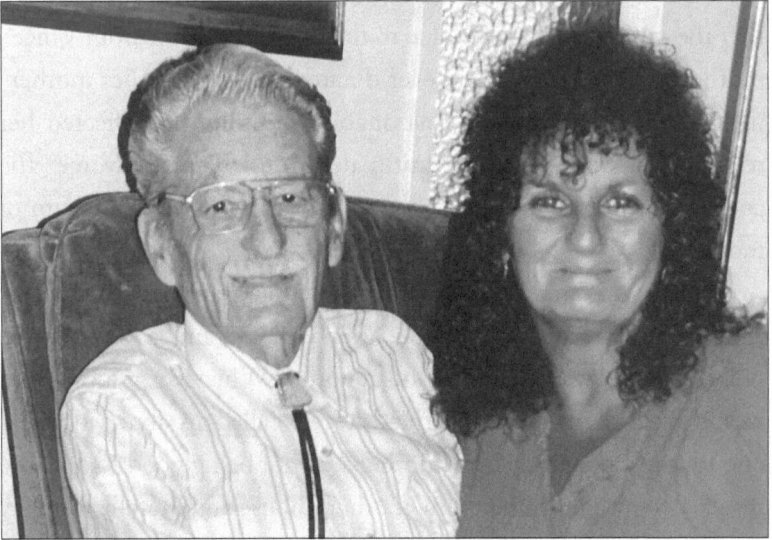

Patsy and Wayne, 1992

SIX

Finding My Niche

One month after I moved in with Gary, I started a new nursing position at a psychiatric facility named Gladman Hospital, about twenty minutes from Gary's apartment. It was not the job I wanted to have long term because the building was in a high-crime area, and because I was still pursuing my legal career. However, it would give me the financial security I needed until I passed the bar and could find a job that would challenge me and stretch my abilities.

One evening, I came out of the hospital at 11:30 p.m. to find my car had been broken into. The driver's side window was smashed, the signal light was torn off the steering wheel, and the glove compartment was left wide open. I felt sick to my stomach. I went to find the hospital guard who was supposed to be watching the parking lot and reported the incident to him, then nervously drove home, unsure of what else they might have done to my car.

This was the second such incident I'd experienced at the hospital—just a few weeks earlier, one of my car tires had been punctured. Gary and I had talked then about whether I should resign, and while I wasn't sure that was the route I wanted to take, just having his support meant so much to me.

A couple of days after my car had been vandalized, Gary and I were enjoying our evening walk around the lake when he stopped and gave me a serious look. "Lilly, I think you need to listen to the universal message you are receiving through the vandalism of your car."

I agreed. I didn't want to keep working in such a dangerous neighborhood; I was fortunate that I hadn't been assaulted.

Gary continued, "I think you should leave that job and focus on studying for the bar exam in July. We're partners, and what affects one of us affects the other. I know you want to work and be financially independent, but you can accomplish this later."

I spent the night thinking about what he said, and the next day I gave my notice to the hospital. I felt a tremendous sense of relief, and I was grateful that Gary was so supportive.

A week later, on Easter Sunday, I got up in the morning to find several boxes sitting on the floor by our sofa. When I asked Gary what they were for, he grinned and said, "Do you want to know now, or after you have had a cup of coffee?"

I was addicted to coffee and was nonfunctional without at least one cup, but I also couldn't stand to wait to open surprise packages. After a brief internal debate, I decided I was willing to forgo the coffee. "Okay, what's in these boxes?"

Gary had me sit down on the sofa and handed me a letter. I opened it to find a thank you note for signing up for the California Preliminary Multistate Bar Exam Review program. In the boxes, I discovered workbooks covering each area of the law that I would be tested on. I was shocked; this program cost about a thousand dollars. Having someone support my education in this way was completely unexpected. My parents had never supported me in my nursing career, either financially or emotionally, and my ex-husband and I had divorced over the fact that I wanted to obtain my nursing degree. I'd worked full time as a nurse to put myself through my law degree, and I was having difficulty passing the bar exam because I continued to work full time to support myself, limiting my ability to study. It felt so wonderful to have someone support my goal and believe in me.

I hugged him and said through my tears, "Thank you so much from the bottom of my heart and soul. I love you so much." This gift meant more to me than I could ever say.

After I got the law books, Gary asked if I would like to join him at the California Trial Lawyers Association board meetings each month. We were both already involved in the CTLA, with him being a past president and me being a former student member of the Los Angeles Trial Lawyers Association. I had joined the CTLA because I knew that it was a great way to meet people and make professional contacts; attending the board meetings would give me the opportunity to develop those contacts even further. So, I agreed.

Gary and I socialized with the other board members and their partners at the dinners after each meeting, and this camaraderie gave me a deeper sense of belonging. I made some very interesting, fun, and intelligent friends whom Gary and I enjoyed spending time with over the ensuing years. I also enjoyed being an "insider" within this powerful group.

Joining these meetings also led to an incredible opportunity for me, which came after the Hill-Thomas hearings in 1991. Anita Hill was called to testify about the character of Clarence Thomas and his fitness to serve on the Supreme Court. Ten years earlier, Hill had become an attorney-adviser to Clarence Thomas in the United States Department of Education and at the Equal Employment Opportunity Commission in 1982. Hill testified that during her employment with Thomas, he had made sexually provocative statements, boasted about his sexual prowess, and described to her acts he'd seen in pornographic films such as rape scenes and bestiality. Despite her testimony, the Senate voted 52-48 to confirm Thomas as an associate justice of the Supreme Court. I, along with many other women, was outraged by this decision.

Public interest in, and debate over, Hill's testimony launched public awareness around the issue of sexual harassment in the United States. The topic was now more openly discussed, though many women still found it difficult to come forward—they would often be blamed for what happened to them or dismissed entirely.

Soon after this event, Gary Paul, the current president of the CTLA, asked me to be chairwoman of a newly established Committee on Gender Bias. As a result of the Thomas-Hill hearings, the association would now be providing a mandatory continuing education program for lawyers on the elimination of gender bias in the legal profession. I would not only chair the committee but also present seminars on this topic. I was honored that he felt I could take on this responsibility and gratefully accepted the offer, happy that I could use my law degree to contribute to the organization.

There were now three programs that lawyers in California were required to attend before their license would be renewed: ethics, substance abuse, and the newly added elimination of gender bias. Gary was teaching ethics while our dear friend Ed Caldwell was teaching substance abuse. One day, as we were driving to court, Gary surprised me by asking if I wanted to join him and Ed in offering a joint program. Instead of lawyers having to do three one-hour sessions, he suggested we create a single three-hour continuing education program. I agreed to join them and found it exciting that we would share this experience together.

Gary, Ed, and I presented these seminars two times a year for about three years. Our first presentation together was nine months after the Hill-Thomas hearings. There were about 150 trial lawyers in the audience, most of them being men, and I was happy to be the last speaker so I could size up the audience and get comfortable with them. It had been several years since I'd last presented a seminar, and the audience at that time had been female nurses. Now I was speaking primarily to men on this brand-new subject of gender bias. I was treading on new territory, so I wasn't sure what responses I might get.

Finally, my turn arrived. Placing a steadying hand on my microphone, I willed a confident smile upon my lips while I waited for my vision to clear. The silence in the room was palpable. My carefully constructed mask slipped for a moment, and I was no longer the grown-up nurse and legal professional. I was simply Lilly Radziewicz, the young girl who battled her insecurities to find a way to believe in herself, even when her mother told her she shouldn't.

I couldn't allow the audience to see me falter in my first talk.

Closing my eyes for a split second, I reached deep within myself to find my faith and vision, knowing Gary and Ed were sitting right behind me. I let the insecure child within me slip away, along with all her worries and aspirations. I then summoned my power, assumed the role of a confident woman with an important message to convey, and began to speak.

I told the audience some of the many stories I'd heard from my female lawyer friends, along with some of my own experiences, about the behavior and attitudes of male lawyers and judges toward women practicing law. I talked about Jackie Taber, a well-known female judge whom I had previously interviewed, and how she could only find a job as a secretary at first even though she was a fully qualified lawyer. I talked about how female lawyers were often referred to as "honey," as a paralegal, or as a secretary by male judges and attorneys when they were representing clients in court. There had even been comments by a judge such as, "I didn't expect to have an attractive lawyer before me today. What is your name?"

I gave examples of the casual yet inappropriate ways men touch women in the workplace, such as a male colleague placing his hand on a woman's shoulder as she walked out of the room or placing his hand on her elbow as she walked toward the elevator. These may seem innocent, but they are intimate behaviors that make many women uncomfortable in a professional setting—ones that would not happen between two male lawyers.

Sharing one of my own experiences, I told them about the day I stopped by my constitutional law professor's office to ask a question about one of his lectures. As I entered his office, he motioned me to sit in the chair in front of his large wooden desk. He was sitting with his legs crossed and outstretched on his desk, and he leaned back in his chair with his hands behind his neck during the conversation. After we discussed my question, he said, "By the way, I have been curious about why you wanted to go to law school. You have a very successful career as a nurse, and if you were my wife, I wouldn't have let you go." I was stunned! I looked straight at him and said, "Well, I am not your wife, and I want to combine my interests in both nursing and law to pursue the area of medical malpractice." Then I thanked him for answering my question, walked out to my car, got inside, and screamed. I was fortunate the semester was coming to an end, and soon I did not have to see or deal with him again.

Presenting these seminars ended up being a very rewarding experience. The audience responded with many comments and questions, showing that this exchange was invaluable to all involved. This was new material for the male lawyers in the room, and the female lawyers finally had a safe place to tell their colleagues what actions and comments were not acceptable to them. While some of the male participants expressed anger after being called out for their sexist attitudes, there were many who thanked me for helping them see their actions from a new perspective so they could understand which ones may be problematic. I was honored to have a platform to help make a difference for both the men and women in my audience.

I was also happy to be making the legal profession more welcoming to women, something that I knew was sorely needed. There were very few women in the legal profession when I first entered law school in 1980—only 20 percent of my class were women. And in 1988, when I decided to join the California Trial Lawyers Association as a student member, only about 10 percent of members were women. I was confident about joining the association because of my success as a nurse; after years of working with surgeons and dealing with their egos, I felt I could hold my own against any man. However, I knew that not every woman had that same confidence. Making the legal profession more accessible to women was going to be a long process, so I was happy to see the world taking baby steps in that direction.

In the fall of 1991, I was offered a position as an adjunct faculty member at the University of San Francisco's School of Nursing and Health Professions, where I'd teach psychiatric nursing for the fall and spring semesters. Since I was still waiting for the results of the bar exam, I decided to accept. I was happy to teach students again, and I loved watching them turn from nervous students into confident nurses.

During this time, Gary was working as a trial lawyer representing plaintiffs who had been involved in serious car accidents, had been wrongfully terminated from their jobs, or had serious injuries as a result of medical malpractice. One day, Gary asked me to look over some medical records to see if there were any discrepancies between their records of the plaintiff and her contentions as opposed to defense's argument against her claims. I had previously worked as an expert witness for psychiatric patients on several occasions and had developed my skills as an expert in this area, so I agreed, and thus I began working for Gary's firm as an independent medical-legal consultant on a part-time basis. Since I was becoming more known in the legal community through my membership with the CTLA, I then began being asked by other lawyers to be an expert witness on cases involving psychiatric patients. As this work expanded, I realized that my dream of combining my interests in nursing and law was evolving better than I'd ever imagined.

After the first year of work with Gary's firm, I went to court with Gary on several cases in a new role. During trials, I would sit next to his clients to offer emotional support and answer any questions they might have about their case. Soon, though, I was able to offer Gary an unexpected benefit to my presence in the courtroom. I wasn't always as compassionate as Gary was, and as a result I could sometimes see the holes in his case and in his argument to the jury. Gary was a strong advocate for his clients, and I respected him for his trial lawyer skills, but sometimes his compassion meant he didn't see everything clearly.

For example, as we were driving home from court one afternoon, Gary asked, "What did you think of the plaintiff today when she was up on the stand?"

I replied with honesty, drawing from my observational skills and my experience in psychiatric nursing. "I didn't believe her, and she didn't come across as being very sincere about her injuries."

My response clearly caught Gary off guard. With anger in his voice, he demanded, "How can you be so hard on her? She's been through a lot of pain, and I did my best to help her explain her story."

I explained to Gary that the way the plaintiff described her injuries was going to make a difference in the way the jury saw her injuries. And because the plaintiff was a woman, I also knew that the jury could be biased against her. I then told him how his client could explain her injuries so they would seem more believable. "During your direct examination of your client, she was nervous and unsure of her answers. She mumbled her words, she was evasive in answering your questions, and she would look down and away from the jury as she spoke. These behaviors made her look like she was lying. She needed to show she was truthful by being strong and direct in her answers, and she needed to look at the jury as she spoke with confidence and certainty."

Noticing the look on Gary's face, I continued, "Look, you asked me to give you my thoughts. If you are going to get angry with me when I offer my opinion, then don't ask me. Let the jury tell you what they think. I just know that if I am noticing these issues, then the jury likely feels the same way." As we continued our drive home, I could see that Gary was considering what I said.

The next day, Gary decided to have his client tell her story in the way I'd recommended, and they won the case. Afterward, Gary questioned the jury about their opinions of his client. They told him they had a hard time believing her during the first day, but upon hearing her story again the next day, they understood what she had gone through.

Through instances like this, I began to gain more credibility with Gary and some of his partners. Gary and I also discovered that we made a good team. He was the ultimate optimist while I was the defense-oriented pessimist and combining these two viewpoints gave us a good perspective on cases.

There was another benefit to me being at his trials. When I was there, I could observe the complex dynamics that go on in a courtroom—the relationships between the lawyer, their client, the judge, the jury, the court reporter, the bailiff, and the defense attorneys. There were so many non-verbal behaviors occurring between all the players on the stage, and if you paid close attention, you could feel these tensions in the courtroom. I enjoyed watching the interplay of all these forces, and because I was there in court with him, I could fully appreciate and understand what his day was like—it's almost impossible to truly understand what goes on in a trial without being there. With me attending his cases, Gary did not have to try and explain how tough his day was.

Finding My Niche

Not every couple enjoys working together, but Gary and I found that doing so pushed us to grow and develop as a couple. It helped that we both wanted to push ourselves, both spiritually and physically, so we could reach our highest potential and be the best we could be. I consider myself fortunate to have found someone whom I can grow with, and whom I can easily spend so much time with.

SEVEN

Meeting Jack Gwilliam

Gary and I were driving from Oakland to Fort Jones, which was on the border of California and Oregon, on a warm summer day in June. He had decided to introduce me to his biological father, Jack, and was visiting him for the first time in two years—Gary's busy work schedule and separation from Liz had made it hard for him to visit. And as he drove, I could tell that something was weighing heavily on his mind.

"Gary, what are you thinking? You seem preoccupied."

Gary explained that he and his father had never had a good relationship. His parents separated when Gary was two years old— apparently, his mother came home from work one day to find Gary in the bathtub and Jack so drunk he could hardly walk or talk. She was livid and told him to get out, and they divorced shortly after this incident. Gary then didn't see his father again for years.

"That must have been a very difficult time for you," I said as I tried to imagine that little boy coping with all this.

"Yes and no. I was too young to remember him, and my mom married Wayne soon after."

"Gary, the first two years of your life were spent with your father and mother. Even if you don't remember that time, it still would have had an impact on you. Do you remember anything about him?"

Gary shook his head. "No. My maternal grandmother didn't like him, and my mother and her two sisters never talked about him again, other than to make negative comments."

After a pause, Gary continued. "The first time I met my dad was when I was eight years old. My mom told me she wanted me to meet Jack Gwilliam, which was how I learned that Wayne was not my father. I was so happy to hear this because I never liked Wayne." They met that first time at Jack's office in Ogden, Utah, but Gary said the conversation between them was stilted and awkward. "My father asked me all kinds of questions about my school, friends, and any interests I had in sports. But I didn't know what to say to my 'real' dad."

As we drove through the small town of Fort Jones, Gary explained that his father had been a very successful insurance and real estate salesman in the 1950s and moved to Glendora, California, while Gary and his mother lived in Seattle. Jack was also one of the founding fathers of Alcoholics Anonymous. Because he was doing so well for himself, Gary's mother suggested that Gary go and live with Jack when Gary was eighteen. He had been getting into trouble at school for smoking pot and was getting in with the wrong crowd, and now that he was graduating from high school, he needed his father's direction. So, ten years after meeting his dad for the first time, Gary moved to California to live with his dad, his stepmother (Helen), and their three daughters (Shana, Lisa, and Linda). Gary went on to Citrus College and won the award for most likely to succeed in his class. Then Jack left Helen and married another woman, leaving Gary to help care for his family.

Gary went on to attend Pomona College, then graduated from Boalt Hall (now the UC Berkeley School of Law) in 1962. His drinking problem began in college but became worse after he got married to his first wife and started to practice law. He did not go to AA like his father did, but he did stop drinking in 1984 after Ed Caldwell and Liz Gwilliam held an intervention. Gary has remained sober ever since.

"I was not close to my father," Gary explained. "I never shared my life with him during either of my marriages. I was so angry with him for not supporting me as a child, and for leaving me to support my stepmother and stepsisters."

Gary then told me that one part of his sobriety journey is making amends and asking forgiveness from the people you have wronged. Part of this was that he needed to let go of his anger toward his father around the way he had abandoned him.

I listened to his history, trying to understand all the relationships. "Gary, I am so happy we are driving to see your dad. I think his eightieth birthday is a wonderful time for you to visit, and I thank you for sharing this special time with me."

"Would you do me a favor?" he asked. "After you meet him, I would really like you to tell me your psychological impression of him." I agreed.

Soon we drove up to a small one-story home with a green and beige exterior. I could feel Gary's anxiety in his constant reassurances that it was okay if I didn't like his father. I did my best to keep an open mind; my own parents were not the easiest people to introduce my partners to either.

When the front door opened, we were met by a stocky man with thinning gray hair. He was sitting in a wheelchair with a nasal cannula running from his oxygen tank—he was suffering from emphysema due to years of heavy smoking—but otherwise he looked great for his age. His skin was smooth, and his blue eyes were bright and alert. Gary introduced us, and Jack said, "It's good to see you again, and to meet Lilly."

Jack's wife, Leila, moved from behind the wheelchair to greet us. She was a short woman in her mid-seventies and wore a plaid dress you'd expect to see on a farm in the 1950s. She gave me a warm, firm handshake, declaring, "So glad to meet you!" As we clasped hands, I noticed that her face was pleasant with warm, friendly blue eyes.

Jack motioned for us to sit at the table and placed himself against the wall. Gary sat across from him while Leila and I took our places next to one another. As we began chatting about work and life over some snacks, I realized that I liked his dad—he seemed genuinely interested in his son.

Wanting to learn more about Gary's past, I said to Jack, "I imagine you had time with Gary when he was young that you may remember, but Gary does not. Do you have any memories that stand out to you?"

Jack laughed heartily. "Oh, yes! We only had one bathroom in the house, and I would spend time in there, reading the paper and shaving. When Gary was about two years of age, he would knock on the door and ask, 'Whatcha doin in there, Dad? Shavin?'"

I looked over at Gary and he smiled; he had never heard this story before. Gary asked, "Dad, did you ever try and get in touch with me during all the years we were apart?"

"Gary, yes, I did. I wrote your mother and grandmother letters to try and set times to see you. But they were angry with me because of my drinking, so they would not answer me." Gary later told me he was not surprised to hear that they had done this to his dad. He knew his maternal grandmother and mother were both strong matriarchs who did not care for men, except for Gary himself.

Leila and I sat off to the side as Gary and his dad continued talking. Jack asked about Gary's work as a trial lawyer, and Gary asked more questions about how his father had tried to get in touch with him over the years. I saw the sadness in both of their eyes as they talked, and Jack was listening to every word Gary spoke with a look of pride on his face. It was as if he were trying to capture all the missed years with every word spoken. I found this situation sad, and tears began softly running down my cheeks. I ignored it at first, but when the time seemed right, I asked, "Could you please get up and hug each other?"

And they did. The love and sadness in the room was palpable, and the tears kept rolling down my face.

On our way back to Oakland, Gary said he felt better after seeing and talking to his dad, then asked me what I thought. I replied, "I enjoyed listening to him, and I think he genuinely wanted to get in touch with you during those early years. I think he still cares about you and would like to establish a relationship if you're willing to forgive him. He's missed seeing you grow up, and since you are his only son, that must have been hard on him. I support whatever decision you make in whether you want to continue seeing your father."

Gary was quiet for some time before he spoke again. "I would like to keep in touch with him, and perhaps send him some money. I know he needs a ramp for the front door to get in and out of the house, and I know they are living only on their social security. I do not want to loan him money, so this would be a gift, because I would like to try and make his life a little easier for the time he has left."

Gary and I went to see Jack and Leila on several occasions over the next three years. We invited them to stay with us in our Oakland apartment to celebrate his father's eighty-first birthday, along with his sister, Shana, her husband, Al, and Gary's three daughters. Jack had never met his teenage granddaughters before that day, and I think this meeting went as well as it could, all things considered.

One day, as the relationship between Gary and his father deepened, we were driving home when Gary said, "You know, in all these years I was never able to call Jack, or any man, 'Dad.'" Gary had tears in his eyes. "I can finally call him Dad now."

Jack Gwilliam died in June 1994. Before his passing, Gary was not only able to forgive his father for not being there in his early life, but also enjoy getting to know his father in his later years and finding his Dad. I was honored to play a role in this story and happy that Gary felt I helped him forgive his father.

Gary also told me over the ensuing years that I'd helped him establish a relationship between his father and his children. They finally got to meet their grandfather at our home, a meeting that was very important to all of them. It was a beautiful unfolding of love that I will always remember.

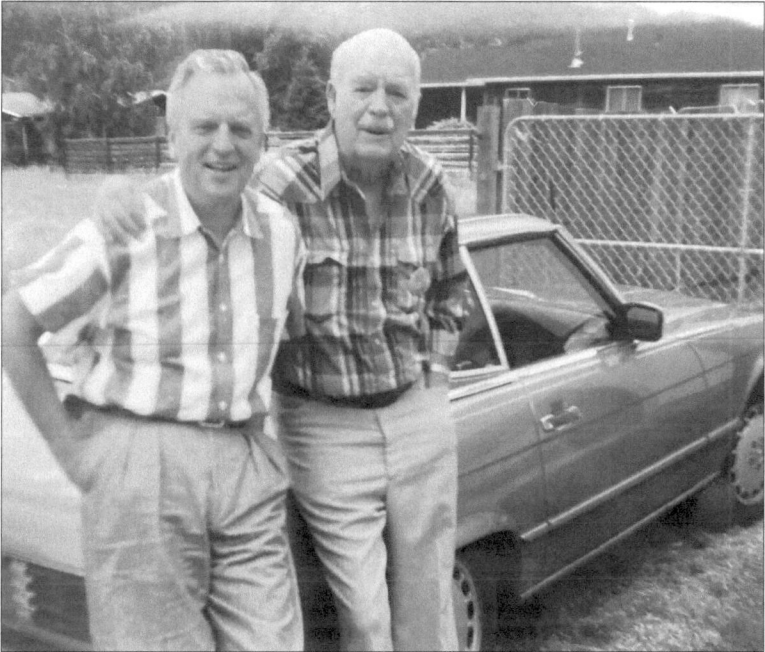

Gary and his "Dad," 1992

EIGHT

Fiji

Gary and I had been together for two years when we met with our lawyer friend GP for brunch on a cold November Sunday. GP was a lawyer who has his own law firm in Fiji along with some family who live in the area. As we sipped our coffee and ate a selection of delicious food, GP told us about the history of his country and his family.

Six years prior, in 1987, there was a coup in Fiji. The Indian residents were quite prominent and successful in business, and the Fijians wanted to overthrow them and get their land and power back. Being of Indian descent, GP decided to move his family to Hayward, California, where they still lived. He maintained his law practice in Fiji and had been a prominent figure in the law society of Fiji, and he traveled back from Fiji to Hayward at least once a month to be with his family.

After this discussion, GP leaned forward with an eager yet uncertain look on his face. "I'd like to invite you both to participate in our fourth Fiji Law Society Convention in July. Gary, you can come up with your own topic to present on, but Lilly, I know you have spoken on gender issues before. Could you speak on the issue of rape? There has been an underground women's movement going on for several years with the goal of helping victims of rape, and we believe that having a speaker from outside of Fiji would add some legitimacy to the topic." He also told us this would be the first time the convention had run since the 1987 coup—membership had dropped significantly during that time, but they had now recovered and had enough interest to restart the event.

Gary and I looked at one another with a big smile, surprised by this invitation. Gary said, "GP, I would be honored to participate in this historic convention."

I agreed. "I would be honored and pleased to talk on such an important topic. I can imagine how sensitive a subject this is for the women of Fiji."

GP went on to explain that in Fiji at that time, rape was considered an offense against public morality instead of an offense against the person. From the onset, the victim must convince the magistrate that she did not consent to intercourse and did not lead her attacker on. The victim also needed to show corroboration, which meant that a witness was needed—something that was almost never possible.

Speaking on this topic in that context seemed like it would be quite difficult, but I liked being challenged. Gary decided his speech would be "Law of Torts: The Trial Practice and the Law."

Our expenses were going be fully paid, so Gary and I decided to ask our children if they would like to join us. Two of his daughters, Catherine and Jen, agreed to come with us, and Gary and I were happy that they could. It would give them an opportunity to spend time together, and Gary and I could have quality time with them as well. Unfortunately, the rest of our children had other commitments and were not able to join us.

Seven months later, we arrived in Fiji and met up with Catherine and Jen at the hotel. Catherine's face was glowing with happiness and wonder as she ran up and kissed her father; she had never been on a vacation with him throughout her twenty-four years and was clearly overjoyed to be here with him now. Jen's long dark hair was pulled back behind her ears, and her brown eyes were shining as she told us how great it was to finally arrive after a fourteen-hour flight from San Francisco.

Soon after, two of the hotel staff came from behind the desk to meet with us. Both women were wearing their national dress, the *sulu*, which resembled skirts and were decorated with beautiful patterns and designs. One woman was tall and slender, wearing a green top with a long green and beige patterned skirt that emphasized her handsome brown face and short dark hair. She smiled and greeted us, then handed me several notes requesting that I appear on a radio show from New Zealand. The other staff member wore a red flower-patterned long dress with short sleeves. Her long black hair was pulled back in a bun. She had a round face with large brown eyes and a warm, welcoming smile. "Dr. Phelan," she said, "please let us know if we can bring anything to your room that will make your visit here more comfortable. We are looking forward to your talk and have been waiting a long time to have someone speak on this issue." What a generous welcome. I found myself a bit overwhelmed as I took in all this good news as well as their gracious attitude.

GP then came to the hotel and told us that several women from the underground women's movement would be attending my presentation. I felt a daunting sense of responsibility to these women and hoped I could live up to their expectations.

After dinner that first night, Gary and I went for a walk along the beach and tried to get a sense of the island. As we walked, we saw many families living in small wooden huts. I noticed the women were doing all the work of preparing dinner outside the huts, cooking over the fire or chopping fruit and vegetables on a table while the young children ran around, half-dressed in the warm, humid weather. The men were gathered in small groups, lying or sitting on the grass with their bottles and glasses of alcohol, laughing or arguing.

As we walked in silence, I wondered how many of the families I was passing by included victims of rape. I had learned from GP that it was common for Fijian women to experience abuse from their husbands and boyfriends, and it appeared to me that the men were used to being catered to by their wives or girlfriends. However, I also considered that what I was seeing wasn't the full picture. I wanted to be careful not to make assumptions based on this very slim slice of Fiji, or to make judgments based on my own American culture.

The day of the conference, I found out that I would be the first speaker at the convention, and the only female speaker from outside of Fiji. I found this a little terrifying, but I pushed those feelings aside. As I stood in the hallway, listening to the buzzing of the audience, I took a deep breath, remembered why I was there, and focused on the message I wanted to convey. Gary gave me a thumbs up as I walked onto the stage to greet the audience made mostly of about one hundred male lawyers. Catherine and Jen were there too, and I could see several women scattered in the audience. I decided I was speaking for them. During my speech, I spoke about how the current common law and legislation meant that rape cases were not likely to result in convictions. It was my belief that there was a need for legislative change, and that we couldn't expect the common law to change until the attitudes toward rape victims changed as well.

I went on to talk about how the myth that "she must have asked for it" was one of the greatest stumbling blocks in rape prosecution. This belief needed to change. Just as open windows in a house didn't justify burglary, a woman's alleged bad character or state of dress doesn't justify rape.

After I finished, the audience applauded, and I could see that Gary was proud of me. The women in the audience also came up and thanked me; I hoped that my words would help with their cause.

After my presentation, I went to lunch with a group of lawyers, both men and women, who told me they thought the presentation was a success. The most memorable discussion I had was with a young woman who had gone to London to attend law school. She said, "I was looking forward to your talk today because I have been working with women who have been abused and raped. It has been stressful, and I have thought about leaving Fiji and returning to London." Her eyes teared, and she could hardly talk. "But as I listened to you, I realized that I must stay here because I now know that this is what I am supposed to do. Thank you." I was so grateful to hear that I'd made an impact on at least one person, and I thanked her for sharing this with me. It was the most powerful and meaningful presentation I'd ever given in my life.

The next day, I was amazed to see that my presentation was described in a local newspaper as an unqualified success, and that it would help society come to grips with everything that was wrong with the Fijian law. Below is a quote from an editorial comment in the *Fiji Post* newspaper on August 2, 1993:

"The paper on rape, delivered by Dr. Phelan, was just one of the many front-on assaults made on issues important to society. Arguably, her views and the resultant commentary may have played a major part in Attorney-General Kelemedi Bulewa reaffirming Government's commitment to review the outdated laws used in Fiji, particularly the law of corroboration which appears to heavily not favour victims of rape."

My reward for the speech I gave came a year later, when one of the lawyers I met at the convention sent me a letter and newspaper article telling me that Fiji had changed the law. The High Court had agreed with the prosecution that a woman should sit as an assessor for a manslaughter trial in which another woman had been killed. In Fiji, assessors provide guidance on community wisdom, expectations, standards, and experiences. This role was exclusively filled by men up until this point, but it was determined that a woman's perspective was needed in this case. This paved the way for obtaining women assessors for rape cases, which would help circumvent some of the prejudices against women. It gave me immense pleasure to know that I had some small part in helping make this island a safer place for the women who lived there for generations to come.

With the convention finished, Gary and I spent the next few days exploring the islands of Fiji with Catherine and Jen. GP enhanced our family trip by being a most gracious host to us. We were invited to his home for an authentic Indian dinner, and we met his two male cousins, who were also law partners, and their wives. They cooked us a wonderful meal of mahi mahi, rice, breadfruit, cassava, vegetables, and taro leaves. It was such a treat to be invited inside of his family life and learn more about them.

Fiji

Each evening, Gary and I would go to a local restaurant with the girls and chat as we listened to the waves rushing up against the beach. It was warm and humid, but it was a delight just to be together. I enjoyed watching Gary with his daughters and loved listening to stories from their childhood.

Catherine spoke rapidly and with enthusiasm on any subject. She'd get animated, and her beautiful brown eyes sparkled as she told us about her day. Jen was more reserved, but it was clear that she enjoyed being with Catherine, and they often laughed together about something amusing that happened that day. For example, when the glass-bottom boat we took to our huts on a smaller island broke down, we had to wait over an hour for another boat to bring us back to our rooms—the drivers of the boats were trying to get in touch with one another to no avail. Luckily, we were not very far from shore, so we just relaxed and looked at all the sea creatures below until help arrived. The girls found this situation to be so funny for some reason, and Gary and I just sat back and enjoyed them being silly. Gary looked at his daughters with love and adoration and openly expressed his feelings of pride. I would sit back with my drink, enjoying the ambience and feeling the love around us.

The four of us spent the next three days exploring nearby islands, walking along the white sand beaches, and dipping our feet in the crystal-clear turquoise water. At night, we enjoyed the mass of stars in the night sky. Sharing of our time together in Fiji was one of the first steps Gary and I took in building our family relationships with Jen and Catherine, and we hoped there would be more times like this in the coming years.

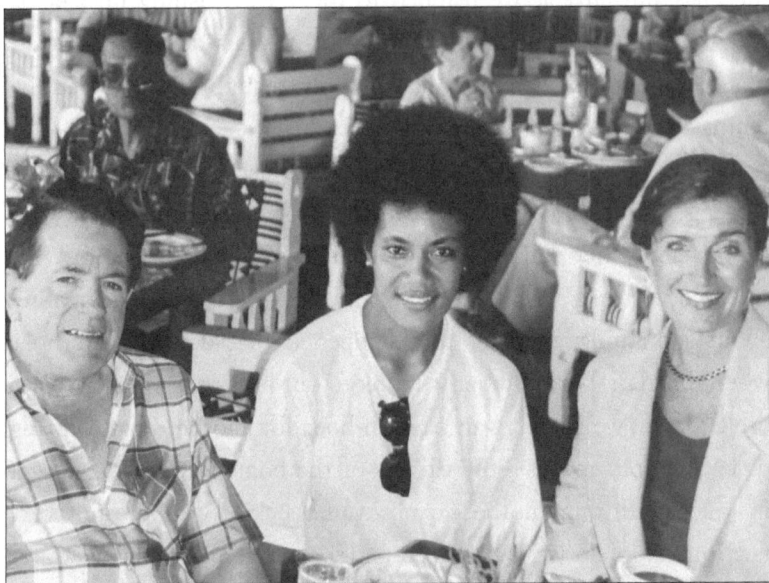

Lilly in Fiji with some local lawyers, 1993

NINE

The Dance of Intimacy

After Gary and I had been together for three years, I decided it was time to call Liz, his soon to be ex-wife. She and Gary had been working through the process of getting divorced, and while she knew about me, we had never met or spoken. However, recent events had made me realize that it was perhaps time for us to talk.

The turning point came when Jen graduated from high school. I'd spent quite a bit of time with her over the past three years, yet I was not invited to her graduation ceremony. It hurt to be excluded from this significant event in Jen's life—I thought that Gary and I were in this for the long term, but being left out like this made me feel like our relationship was being treated as something temporary and unimportant. I later learned there were many conflicted reactions, fueled by grief, that contributed to this decision.

On the day of the graduation ceremony, I wanted to be excited for Gary, yet all I could feel was a sense of exclusion and pain. I gave my congratulations to Jen over the phone and wished Gary a wonderful time, then took a long walk around Lake Merritt to walk off my sadness. I felt so vulnerable and so insecure about my relationship with Gary, and even though he was wonderfully supportive of me and our relationship, I wondered where we stood.

At first, once we got past the event, I did my best to take the high road and just move on. I really tried to use my psychiatric nurse background to help me look at this situation objectively and remove my emotions and insecurities from the equation. I tried to remember that Gary and his family were still grieving the loss of the family they once had, and that there is no time limit for such grief. On the other hand, I struggled to shake the feeling that our relationship was faltering. I finally talked to Gary about my feelings, and he helped me realize there had been a lot of emotional and physical changes since he and I met, and that adjusting to this new reality was challenging for all of us. He and Liz were doing their best to make Jen a priority during her graduation, even if it meant making difficult decisions. This helped me feel better, but it also made me realize that it was time for Liz and I to get to know each other so we could move past this awkwardness and better navigate these family dynamics.

I'd often thought about what I would say to Liz about myself and my relationship with Gary. Was there a right or wrong way to approach your partner's ex-wife? Was there anything I could say that would have any meaning to her? She and Gary had been married for nineteen years; how does one overcome the loss of a spouse after so much time together, if at all? While I had also gotten divorced, I was the one who had ended the relationship, so I couldn't relate to her on that level. I knew I wanted to talk with her, but I didn't know what I should do or say. It was like climbing a mountain for the first time without the necessary equipment—I just had to follow my intuition.

One afternoon, I decided to tell Gary about my plan to call Liz and ask for his thoughts on the matter. His only response was "I cannot imagine you and Liz talking with each other." Otherwise, he did not have a strong opinion. He didn't stop me from calling her, but he didn't encourage me either, nor did he give me any ideas about what I might say to her.

Finally, I decided to take the plunge and call Liz. While I still wasn't sure what to say, I hoped that we might find some common ground.

When Liz picked up, I explained who I was and asked her if she would like to have coffee with me. In a calm voice, she replied, "I would be happy to talk with you over the phone rather than meet for coffee." I was relieved that she was willing to speak with me at all.

Liz went on. "I've heard about you from Gary's partners and their wives, and of course from the girls. I have heard nothing but good things, and I'm happy about that. As you may know, I was shocked to hear that Gary was involved with you just six weeks after our separation. I didn't know whether you knew one another before then or not, so it was quite an adjustment. I want you to know that I've come to understand that you were not the cause of our separation. I've also heard from one of the partners that they wished they could say something negative about you, but they couldn't, and this says a lot." It was good to know that she didn't harbor any ill will toward me; I now felt much more confident about talking with her.

We continued our conversation, getting to know each other better, and I was surprised to find that we could talk with ease and comfort—I could see why Gary loved her. I shared my professional background with her and told her about my own children. Liz told me that she wished she'd developed a career for herself and how satisfying it was when she completed her degree from St. Mary's a few years ago. She now wanted to find a job that she would enjoy and would challenge her.

Liz also told me about her relationship with Gary—their early life together and some of the painful times they went through. I appreciated that she was able to be so open with me, and that she felt comfortable sharing such details.

After talking for about an hour, we both agreed to keep in touch with one another and work together to create an inclusive relationship for the girls. I learned so much from this conversation, and I sensed that we'd established the beginnings of a relationship between us. It was wonderful that we had "met," and I was happy not just for myself but also for Gary and their daughters, Lisa and Jen. It was important to have an open and clear communication between all of us so we could create a loving and supportive environment.

I told Gary about our conversation, and he said it was hard to believe that we'd talked for an hour. I could see pride and delight in his eyes, along with a deeper recognition of who I was. I knew he was happy that I had connected with Liz, and that the two of us were able to get along.

Several months later, Gary and Liz were deciding what Gary might want to keep from the house they'd owned together, and they invited me to join them as he did a final walk-through of the home. I was pleased that Liz now trusted me enough to be a part of these decisions. This would be the first time I met her in person, and I looked forward to seeing her.

Gary and I drove up into the Oakland Hills on a sunny fall afternoon. I had listened to Gary and his daughters talk about their lovely childhood home and how much fun they all had there together—I could only imagine how many more stories the family had to tell.

As we entered the small red brick courtyard that served as the entrance to the home, Gary and I were met by Sam, Gary's favorite dachshund. Liz had kept Sam after the separation, but I know Gary's affection for him had never diminished. While it was clear Sam was happy to see Gary, he was definitely a barker and a protector of the home, so his greeting was quite noisy.

Hearing all the commotion, Liz opened the front door and welcomed us inside. She was a petite woman with short light-brown hair and brown eyes. It was interesting how physically different we looked, though we were only six months apart in age. In my talk with Liz, we had laughed about the fact that he at least did not choose a woman twenty to thirty years younger like a lot of his divorced colleagues had done.

Gary formally introduced us, and Liz graciously offered me a cup of tea. She then proceeded to show me around the house, and as she did so, she told Gary he was free to take whatever was meaningful to him. Gary responded that while he was happy to have the opportunity to make sure he did not leave anything behind, he had all he needed.

I looked around the home that Gary had loved, the place where he had lived with his family, and I felt a sense of sadness. Liz was very gracious, but I knew this moment had to be very hard for her.

After the tour, the three of us sat in the living room as Liz and Gary talked about the finalization of their divorce. I noticed Liz's face had become drawn in sadness, and that Gary seemed sorrowful as well. After a while, I said, "I feel so sad, can you both please stand up and hug each other? It is okay that you both love one another even now." They both rose up and put their arms around each other, breaking into laughter afterward.

Within a few weeks after this meeting, Liz found her niche doing team building seminars for corporations. She became involved in a relationship with a wonderful man not long after that, and we could see how happy she was. Gary and I enjoyed seeing Liz and her friend at various events, and any tension that may have existed between us was replaced with ease and enjoyment. This was especially true at Lisa's college graduation, which was followed by a fun and enjoyable dinner with Liz's brother and Lisa's boyfriend. I was so glad to be a part of this important celebration.

TEN

Exploring My Past

In 1995, Gary and I landed in London for the first leg of our tour through Europe—a five-week journey that would take us from London to Poland, Rome, Florence, and Venice. We had always talked about taking trips like this together, and now, after a year of planning, we were finally here. This was my first trip to Europe, and it seemed like a dream—perhaps because I was still woozy from the broken sleep we got on the plane.

Gary had been to England several years prior, and he used his knowledge of the area to plan interesting places for us to stay and visit. We arrived at 10:30 a.m. London time, and after going through customs and getting our bags, we were met by a driver from the Lanesborough Hotel, where we would be staying. As we were driven from the airport to downtown London, I felt like I was home. My maternal grandfather's family was from England and had been quite prosperous in the ship building industry for several generations. Although my grandfather was born in the United States, I'd always wanted to come to England to see where his family came from.

We drove up to a large four-story white brick building with Bentley cars lined up in the circular driveway. Staff in red uniforms opened our car door and greeted us as we stepped out onto a red carpet that led to the hotel entrance. They then grabbed our luggage and brought us to our room, taking us through a lobby with high ceilings, wood paneling, and red and gold chairs arranged around the reception desk. It was an unbelievable start to our trip. This hotel was especially interesting and significant to me as a nurse as it had been a hospital up until two years prior. After the hospital had closed down, it had been given a new life as an elegant and charming hotel.

The next day, we went on a private tour around the city of London and visited popular tourist sites like Buckingham Palace, Parliament, Piccadilly Circus, Trafalgar Square, and Westminster Abbey. I had heard so much about these places over the years, and I enjoyed being here to experience them for myself. I especially enjoyed visiting the house where Florence Nightingale, an English social reformer and the founder of modern nursing, had lived and died.

Another day, we went to dinner at a local pub followed by watching *Sunset Boulevard*, a musical by Andrew Lloyd Webber about the silent screen era. The story followed Norma Desmond, an aging and forgotten actress, as she dreams about returning to the big screen from her dilapidated mansion in Hollywood. It was both haunting and sad.

For our last night in London, Gary and I decided to have dinner at the Celeste Restaurant, which was attached to the Lanesborough Hotel. It was a richly decorated dining room with a domed glass roof which glowed seductively under the softly lit chandeliers. I wore a simple black dress with black pearls, and my hair was rolled up in a pin-up style that was popular in the forties—elegant but simple. Gary wore a white shirt with a collar and cuffs that had a multi-colored design that accentuated his blue eyes.

During our romantic dinner, we held hands and talked about the events of the day. Gary said, "I love being with you, and I'm happy you are enjoying your trip here in London. I love your excitement about being here."

"How can I not be so happy with you?" I responded. "Gary, this trip is just beginning, and I am already awed by your perfect planning. It has been a dream come true." We looked at one another with the same kind of love and passion that we felt on our first date. In the background, we could hear the song "All I Ask of You" from *The Phantom of the Opera*. It was the perfect end to a perfect day.

Our next stop was Buckland Manor. As we made our way there, we enjoyed a delightful day of driving through the English countryside, stopping by Oxford and having tea in a village along the way.

Buckland Manor is situated in a peaceful and secluded setting, tucked away in an unspoiled area of the Cotswolds. When we arrived, we entered a long gravel driveway with towering trees on both sides and rode toward a large chalet surrounded by colorful manicured gardens. The manor itself, which dated back to the thirteenth century, looked like several Tudor-style houses that had been joined together. As we entered the inner hall to check in, I noticed a paneled sitting room with red and tan slip covers on the sofa and side chairs, which added warmth to the room. A large brick fireplace created a timeless atmosphere, and several vases of multi-colored flowers had been placed on the dark ebony side tables. It felt so serene.

The manor had ten bedrooms, each with their own bath and a fireplace. There were no keys to our room, which was a delightful surprise—it felt like staying in someone's home instead of a hotel. I assumed they vetted their guests for safety, or at least I hoped they did.

As we closed the door to our room, Gary and I took a moment to look around and take it all in. The large four-poster bed was draped in red and gold brocade covers, with mountains of pillows of all shapes and sizes. There was a chest of drawers that looked like it was crafted from solid ebony, a small table, and a lounge chair covered in exquisite embroidery. We pulled back the silk drapes to reveal French windows that looked out over the tree-lined driveway. The room was breathtaking, as were the immaculate flower gardens that stretched out before us.

"Wow, Gary," I said. "I could get used to this style of living."

He smiled. "I'm happy you like it. You deserve to be spoiled."

Each morning, we enjoyed our English breakfast and discussed our sense of having shared past lives—a feeling that had been stimulated by coming to this area. One afternoon, during a tour of a castle in Wickford, I felt a strong connection to a painting done of a young squire. The squire wore black shoes with silver buckles as well as a red jacket with gold shoulder decorations. I had brought with me a St. John red knit suit that had similar aspects to the one in the painting, which made it fun to try and imagine having a prior life here.

Similarly, Gary told me that he'd had a very powerful experience when he'd visited Kenilworth Castle in 1982. He'd felt he was an outsider, as if he'd been in a battle there. When we visited that same castle during our trip, I felt like I'd lived there—like I belonged. It felt like home. There's no way to know the validity of these feelings and experiences, but either way, we enjoyed imagining these past lives.

One week later, we arrived in Poland, the land of my paternal grandparents. I was the only person in my father's family—including his seven brothers, one sister, and all their children—to visit this country. I felt very fortunate that I was able to be here on the land of my forefathers, and I will always treasure my experiences here, which I have been able to share with my children, grandchildren, and Polish cousins who have not yet been able to visit this beautiful and interesting country. Gary was also excited to be here—he had read the book *Poland* by James Michener, and it had made him as enthusiastic to visit this country as I was.

Our first stop was the city of Krakow, which is one of the most beautiful and quaint cities in Europe, surrounded by high brick walls built in the eleventh century. The lifestyle was such a contrast to what we had seen in England, and hearing the Polish language brought back heartwarming memories of my grandparents—I'd always loved listening to them speak in their native tongue.

When Gary and I arrived at the hotel, we were given a small room with two single beds. It was basic, more like a Motel 6 than the lavish hotels we had been staying in, but it was comfortable enough and we slept well, especially since we were tired from our travels.

The next day we went to see the Wawel Royal Castle and the main square (Rynek Główny), which overlooked the Vistula River. We spent the morning walking around and looking at the shops and churches, enjoying the quaint streets and historic buildings along the way. We were impressed by the Gothic church spires that loomed above a patchwork of baroque Romanesque buildings. Walking around the ancient city was an adventure of its own.

Gary and I decided to stop for lunch in the square. As we slowly moved through a long line to get food, I noticed two gentlemen talking at a nearby table. The younger gentleman was reading a book I'd read and loved: *Zen and the Art of Motorcycle Maintenance* by Robert M. Pirsig, a story about man's search for meaning.

I could not help myself. Unsure if the man even spoke English, I smiled and asked, "How are you enjoying the book?"

Surprisingly, he answered, "I am really enjoying it."

"It's one of my most favorite books."

The man responded, "I'm here with my brother. Do you want to join us?"

I was pleased to be invited and felt like I was home, again—how strange to feel so at home in such diverse places. The man, who was in his mid-thirties with blond hair and blue eyes, introduced himself as Stanislaw Obirek. He was a Jesuit priest who taught at Jagiellonian University, which was the oldest university in Poland and one of the oldest in Europe, and he offered Gary and me a private tour of the building the next day.

Stanislaw was born in Krakow and told us about what it was like growing up in Poland. We learned that Krakow was not bombed during World War II, so many of the streets and architecture remained like they were before the war. It was also one of the most important administrative cities of the Third Reich. The Nazis turned Krakow into a German city, and the Jews were confined into over-crowded ghettos before later being deported to Auschwitz-Birkenau and other concentration camps.

One morning, as Gary and I were eating breakfast at our hotel, we heard a voice over a loudspeaker directing the guests who signed up for the Auschwitz tours to move to the lobby of the hotel. The voice sounded exactly like the voice on the loudspeaker in movies like *Sophie's Choice* and *Schindler's List*, and the haunting sound gave me chills. I remembered that we were in a city where the Jewish people were sent to their deaths at a camp just two hours away, and the sorrow and pain felt so real that they were hard to let go of.

The next day, the three of us met again at the café. As we ate, we learned more about our new friend. Stanislaw shared that he too was an educational leader in his family, and he had published several books. He gifted Gary and me two of his books with a meaningful note inside each one, and we would go on to exchange educational material with him for several years.

After a delightful morning with Stanislaw, we had a long, full day of sightseeing. Gary and I then both needed some quiet time, so we had a peaceful dinner together and relaxed to absorb the wonderful experiences we'd had since arriving in Krakow.

We spent our last day touring southern Poland. We drove to the mountains and appreciated how green and colorful the country was. We visited two castles where we enjoyed seeing the lavish lifestyles of Polish kings and were impressed by the history of the country. On our way back to our hotel, we drove by a factory that appeared in *Schindler's List*. We'd decided not to visit Auschwitz because it was further away, and because it would be depressing.

Later that evening, we had a dinner of borscht soup and *pierogi*, a popular Polish cuisine filled with meat, sauerkraut, and mushrooms. This meal reminded me of the dinners my grandmother cooked when I was a young girl. I felt nostalgic at the thought of my grandparents, and as we enjoyed our meal, I looked out over the countryside and realized how much I loved this place. I could only imagine how difficult it must have been for my grandparents to leave this beautiful country and everyone they loved to go to Germany via the underground railroad to escape the Russians. It was an incredibly important and heartwarming trip for me, and it gave Gary a chance to explore and learn more about some of my own history.

Our next destination was Warsaw, and we traveled there via a first-class train ride from Krakow so we could savor the landscape. When we got to the train station, though, we quickly realized that we were lost. We didn't speak Polish, and when we asked where we should go to get the train, we got the same blank look over and over again.

"Gary, this is not good," I said. "We cannot read the signs, and there is no one to help us."

He shrugged his shoulders. "I know, I don't know what to tell you."

We continued dragging our heavy luggage around as we tried to find our way through this maze of a train station. Trains were coming and going, but we didn't know which one was going to Warsaw.

We must have looked lost, because a gentleman finally came up to us and asked if he could help. He was a tall man, about fifty years of age, and he was traveling alone. We were so relieved that he spoke English, and when we told him of our predicament, he told us to follow him as he was also going to Warsaw. We could not have felt more gratitude toward him, and we were pleased to do whatever he said.

The man led us to the first-class coach, where we had our own four-seater cabin with a sliding door for privacy. He then told us that he was in third class but indicated that he would be happy to join us. I was initially uncertain that I wanted to spend the three-hour ride with this stranger, but since we were both very grateful for his help, we invited him to stay.

This man introduced himself as George—though the business card he gave us revealed that this was an anglicized version of his name, Jerzy Przeździecki—and he turned out to be an interesting man. He was an author and playwright living in Warsaw, where he'd grown up. His wife had been a prima ballerina but had retired due to a heart condition, and they had a twenty-one-year-old daughter who was a law student. He had also been previously married and had two sons from his first marriage. It was an unbelievable start to a very engaging conversation. We talked about marriage, books, relationships, Poland, and life in general. When we arrived at our destination, we shared a taxi into town. George then said he wanted to take us on a tour of the city the following day and invited us to dinner so we could meet his wife and daughter.

The next morning, we met George for our private tour of Warsaw. I loved the city immediately. Located on the banks of the Vistula River, it's the capital of Poland and the largest city in the country. As we walked through Old Town, we observed the colorful buildings that had a similar architecture to the ones in Krakow—a wonderful contrast to the modern glass skyscrapers downtown. The scenery was breathtaking, and the energy of the city was palpable.

This city was not at all what I expected. The shops in Warsaw were modern, and the style of dress was very similar to what people wore in the United States. I had an image of their clothes being rather simple and plain, as we'd seen in movies that depicted this city in another era—not the sophisticated and modern looks that I was seeing now.

We went to a museum in the middle of Old Town, and Gary and I were most impressed by a video they had about how the Poles restored Warsaw after the Nazis bombed the city. I had tears in my eyes as I watched how the people used historic paintings, drawings, photographs, and tiny fragments from the ruins—all of which had to be hidden away in secret underground archives—to restore this beautiful city to what it was before the destruction. I felt a swell of pride at being of Polish descent.

This tour was followed by a heartwarming evening with Eva, Claudia, and George. We all sat in their lovely living room, which was small but comfortable, munching on cheese and crackers and enjoying a glass of red wine. I immediately felt a strong connection to this family—especially the daughter, Claudia, with whom I shared an interest in law. Eva told me about her career as a ballet dancer, and Claudia was excited about attending law school. When we went to leave, Claudia became tearful, and we hugged each other. We stayed in contact for a few years after this meeting but unfortunately lost touch.

On our last day in Warsaw, I called my Uncle Julie in New York, the only living relative on my father's side of the family. I had talked to him many times about our family history, and I could tell that he was so pleased I'd called him from Poland.

This trip taught me how valuable travel is on so many levels. On a relationship level, Gary and I learned how well we traveled together. Everything we did was easy and smooth. We enjoyed experiencing new cities and people, and we had similar interests in tourist attractions. We learned so much about each other and saw one another through a new lens. Sharing his love and excitement for life is a gift that I will not take for granted.

On a personal level, the experience of traveling provided a wonderful education that I'd never appreciated before now. The people we met enriched our lives, and we felt a stronger connection to both Krakow and Warsaw because of them. We were privileged to meet such incredible people who were willing to share a part of their lives with us. I also felt more connected with my own family history, and I'm grateful that I was able to share that with Gary.

ELEVEN

Italy

G ary and I traveled from Warsaw to Rome to meet our children for our next adventure. None of our kids had been to Europe before, so we had decided to invite them to join us for two weeks in Italy. We figured a trip like this would provide a neutral ground for everyone to get to know each other better. Lisa was unfortunately unable to come due to other commitments, but Catherine, Jen, Pat, and Liz were all flying in. Gary and I arranged to be there a day ahead of everyone so we could get settled before meeting them at the airport.

We arrived at the Antico Albergo del Sole al Pantheon, a lovely fifteenth-century hotel located on the Piazza della Rotonda, and we could not believe this charming hotel was in the center of so much activity. There were quaint shops around the Roman court along with several cafés with people eating dinner at round tables. I noticed a sense of excitement in the air along with the sound of laughter from the crowd and the hustle and bustle of waiters trying to please their customers.

Gary and I were met by the hotel staff in a small but lovely reception area. After checking in, we entered our room and were delighted to see a carved wood headboard along with a beautiful wood design at the foot of the bed. The sofa was a light gold color that matched the drapes on the window. Our room overlooked the large fountain in the center of the square as well as the Pantheon on the other side of it. As we unpacked, we looked up at our ceiling and saw wood carvings with designs made up of flowers, birds, and the faces of angels. And, as was typical in Europe, there was a very tiny bathroom. It was a beautiful room, with a prime location that we thought would make it easy to explore the city. We decided to have a lovely candlelight dinner at one of the cafés outside our hotel before tucking in for the night.

In the morning, after our delicious buffet breakfast in the hotel courtyard, we walked over to visit the Pantheon. It was a large, windowless structure, built between AD 118 and AD 125, with an oculus at the top of the dome that allowed light into the open room. It also allowed rain inside the Pantheon, but there were twenty-two well-hidden holes in the gently sloped floor to drain the water away. We learned that this temple was dedicated to all the gods of pagan Rome, and it contained the tomb of the famous artist Raphael as well as several Italian kings and poets. Visiting this historical site was a great way to pass the time as we waited for our children to arrive.

Pat, Liz, and Jen all flew in together, and we anxiously awaited their arrival. Unfortunately, they experienced a six-hour delay in New York due to problems with their airplane, so they were quite weary by the time they arrived. My thirty-year-old son, Patrick (Pat P), looked wiped out in the photo we took, with just a faint smile. He wore his baseball hat above his half-shaven face, and his red shirt was open at the neck. His carry-on hung heavily from his right shoulder. My twenty-seven-year-old daughter, Liz, had a big smile and her hands on her hips, as if to say she was here to party! Jen, now nineteen years old, was carrying her passport in her left hand and throwing her heavy bag over her right shoulder with some difficulty. Her tired face made her look like she didn't want to talk to anyone, but a big smile emerged by the time the limo service arrived to take us to our hotel.

Catherine, now twenty-five, flew in separately from Seattle with her boyfriend, who was also named Patrick (Pat M). By coincidence, both Pats were about the same age and height, with dark brown hair and brown eyes. Even their personalities were similar—they were reserved, attentive, fun, and easy to be around.

Everyone was awed by the hotel and its proximity to the Pantheon. Liz and Jen were sharing a room since they'd spent some time together in Oakland. Pat P had his own room, and Catherine and Pat M were in the room next to us. It was so wonderful to have everyone so close together.

During the day, we would all walk around the city of Rome, spending about 90 percent of our time together. Thankfully, we all got along so well! The weather was hot, getting up to a stifling 105°F, so the highlight of our day was having some gelato to cool us down. During dinners and into our evenings together, we would talk about our day's activities and our lives so we could learn more about one another.

One evening I encouraged the kids to share where they had gone to college and what they were currently doing in their lives, and it was fun to see the variety in their interests and experiences. Pat P had an MBA from New York University and was currently working as a controller with a bank in Marin, California. Liz was a second-year graduate student in social work at Adelphi University in New York, and she also worked part-time helping patients at a community care center. Jen was a second-year student at Grossmont College in San Diego, currently enjoying the student life without a clear picture of where her studies would take her. Catherine had graduated from Portland State University in Oregon with a Bachelor of Arts, but she also didn't have a clear direction of what she wanted to do. She was currently working summers at Nordstrom and pursuing a technical writing certificate. And Pat M was working in computer sales.

Gary and I enjoyed seeing Catherine and Pat M together. Pat M was reserved yet easy to be around, always open to learning more about the person in front of him, while Catherine was very social and enjoyed talking about many different topics, especially health. They balanced each other very well.

During our time in Rome, we visited some of the major landmarks including the Colosseum, St. Peter's Basilica, and the Sistine Chapel. We'd all go briefly off on our own, then come back together with the group so we wouldn't miss the next tourist stop. We were all in sync with each other. It was wonderful for Gary and me to see how well our kids were getting along, even while combating jet lag and following such an active itinerary.

After five days in Rome, we hired a van that took us on a tour of Pompeii. This city is famous for being destroyed when Mount Vesuvius erupted in AD 79, covering it in ash and other volcanic debris. The city was preserved for centuries before its ruins were discovered in the late sixteenth century. We all were fascinated by the wonderful wall paintings and mosaics depicting ancient Roman life. It was amazing how these beautiful paintings were once buried with the rest of the city, and that they had been so well-preserved that we were able to enjoy them today.

We ended our day in Florence, checking in at our next interesting accommodations. The Hotel Loggiato dei Serviti was a sixteenth-century building that was part of the stunning Renaissance-era complex. The arches and columns on the exterior of the building created a feeling of grandeur that was mirrored by the beamed ceilings and parquet floors inside. This hotel was once a monastery and had many of the original features, including cross-vaulted ceilings and stone staircases. The rooms were filled with antiques, and each room had a chair and table with fresh flowers. The bathrooms were so small that the toilet was in the shower, which we all had a good laugh about.

In this hotel, Pat P, Liz, and Jen shared a suite. The girls were upstairs in a loft while Pat had his own bedroom on the main floor of the suite, and we could see that they all seemed to get along well.

Our last day trip was to Sienna, a city in Tuscany with narrow streets flanked by medieval brick buildings. The fan-shaped central square, Piazza del Campo, is the site of the Gothic town hall and a fourteenth-century tower that boasts incredible views from its distinctive white crown. This city was a hub for commerce and banking in the thirteenth and fourteenth centuries, and it was fun to imagine the hustle and bustle of this city in its heyday.

While we were walking down those narrow streets, Gary and I took the time to appreciate the delightful family scenes unfolding in front of us. We smiled at the kids laughing and talking together so naturally. Liz and Jen would wander off to take photos of one another, and if one of them found something of interest, they'd shout out to the others to come and see it too. I also loved seeing Pat P and Liz enjoying each other the way they did while they were children—since they no longer lived in the same city, their time together was limited. During this trip they shared memories from their childhood, like how our cat Panther used to love climbing up on top of the kitchen cabinets and looking down at us like she was the queen of the house. It was delightful to see Pat show off his sense of humor and Liz be her usual sharp-witted self.

This trip really helped all of us come together as a family. Gary was wonderful with both Pat and Liz, including them in his plans and asking their opinions on what we should do. I enjoyed listening to Jen and Catherine talk about stories from their childhood, including some about Gary. We all learned more about one another, and we all grew closer as a result.

For our last dinner together, we all decided to get dressed up. Gary and the two Pats wore jackets and ties with nice slacks while the girls and I wore cocktail attire with heels and some simple but elegant earrings. We shared a gourmet dinner together at the Villa San Michele, located high in the hills of Florence, where we had a private room with a round table surrounded by soft amber walls and several flowered plants. We had an amazing view of the rich, green Tuscan countryside, with twinkling city lights and mountains in the background. It was the perfect ending to our time together—a trip we'll always remember with love and fondness.

Gary and I could not have asked for a better blended family vacation. It was our first step toward creating a full family experience that we hoped would continue to develop through the years to come.

Italy

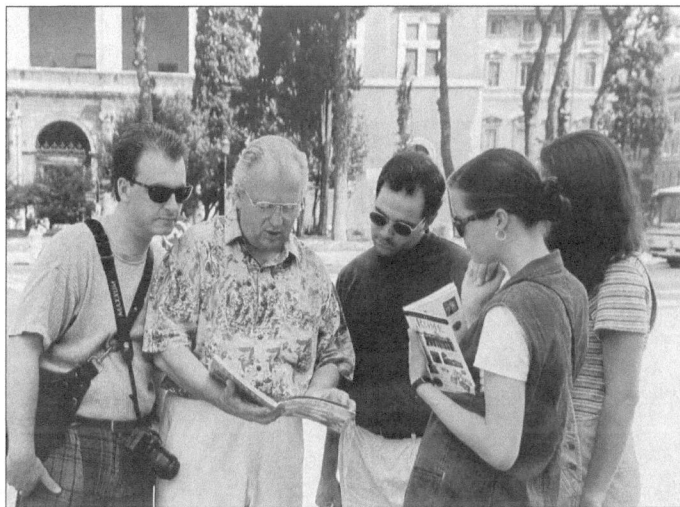

Gary with the kids in Italy, 1994

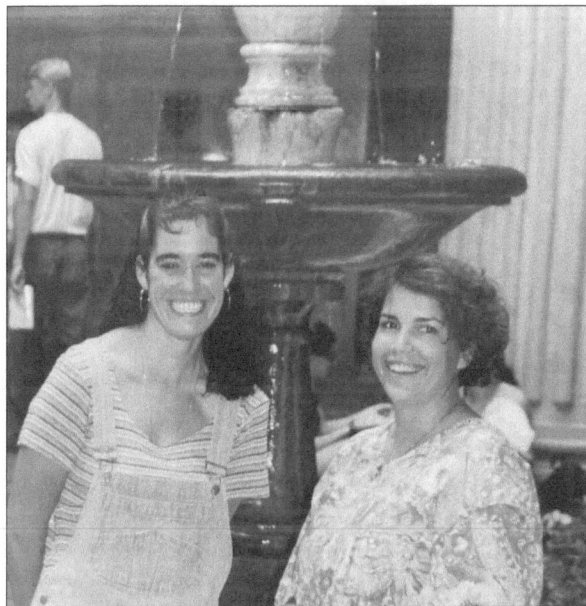

*Liz and Jen in
Italy, 1994*

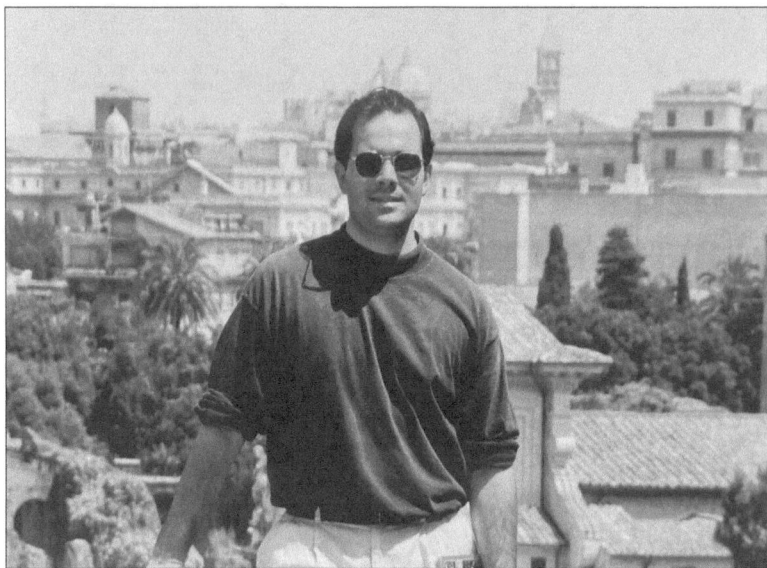

Pat P in Italy, 1994

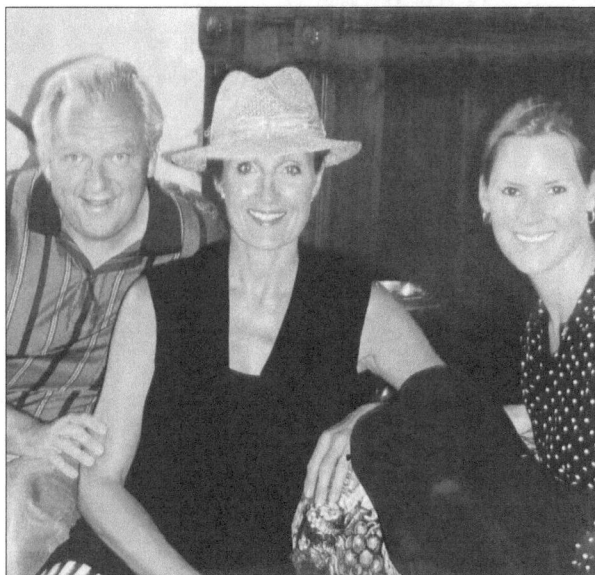

*Gary, Lilly,
and Catherine
in Italy, 1994*

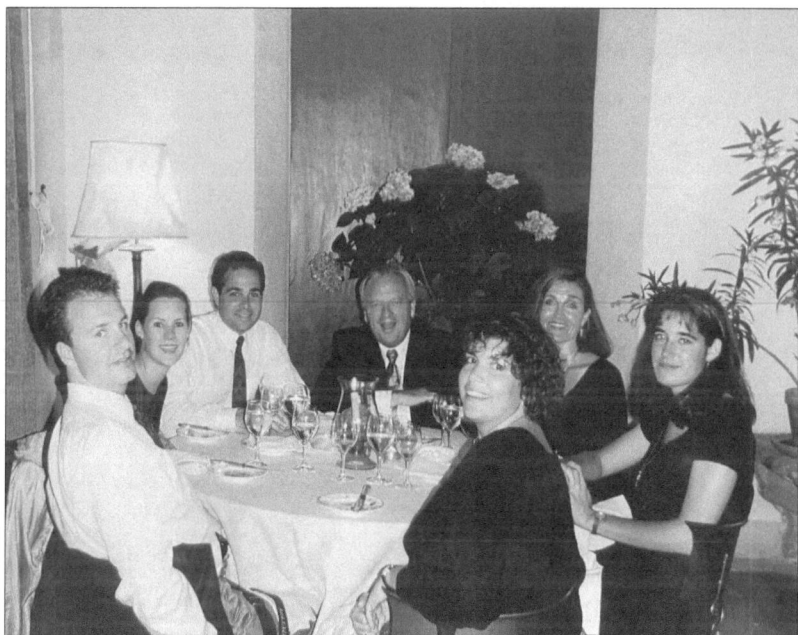

Last dinner in Italy, 1994

TWELVE

Venice

After seeing our children off, Gary and I arrived in Venice, the last city on our magical European trip. There are no cars allowed in the city, which is made up of pedestrian walkways and canals, so a private water taxi took us to our accommodations at The Gritti Palace.

As the taxi toured the waterways on the way to our hotel, I took in the sights of this romantic city. It was early in the evening, and the weather was pleasantly warm. The historic buildings along the Grand Canal, which date back to the eleventh century, were like nothing I'd ever seen before. I was amazed by their bright colors and the unique style of architecture. I later learned they were from the thirteenth to seventeenth centuries and possessed the original Byzantine decorative patterns.

The driver pointed out the Rialto Bridge, which spans the Grand Canal with elegantly curved marble arches. We got off there and wandered through the Rialto Market, then explored part of the canal on foot. There was so much to see in this magical city. I was suddenly overwhelmed with emotion and began to cry—I felt like I was home, and I experienced an unexpected feeling of passion.

Gary noticed my tears and asked, "Are you okay?"

I felt so foolish; I had no idea why I was crying. I reached over to squeeze Gary's arm. "Yes, I'm just overwhelmed by this magnificent city," I said, unsure of how to explain what I was feeling.

We arrived at our hotel through a discrete back entrance, away from the crowds. The lobby was so reminiscent of the old world, with artworks and antiques everywhere, that I felt like I was transported to another place and time. This luxury palace was built in the fifteenth century, and it had been a private residence to noble families for centuries afterward. Our room had two glass doors with sheer curtains and floor-to-ceiling burgundy side drapes. These doors opened out to a small balcony that overlooked the Grand Canal, where we could see the Basilica di Santa Maria della Salute. The bed was decorated in red and gold tones with several small pillows. An antique desk and chair, along with artwork depicting landscapes and famous noblemen, fit with the old-world decor. It was small and cozy, yet we felt like we were in heaven.

Gary and I later learned this enchanting hotel had entertained famous guests like Ernest Hemingway, Elizabeth Taylor, Richard Burton, Greta Garbo, and Brad Pitt, among others. We felt like we were in good company!

After dinner, we strolled alongside the crisscrossing canals and enjoyed the amazing historic architecture of the churches, museums, and restaurants in St. Mark's Square—one of the most interesting places I had ever seen. We both were awed by St. Mark's Cathedral, with its pointed archways, turrets, and figures decorating the roof.

Venice

It is one of the amazing monuments in Europe. The bronze doors came from Byzantium in the eleventh century, and the side entries were rich with mosaics. It was fascinating to know these palaces and buildings had been built on marshland so many centuries ago.

Interesting shops displayed a variety of carnival masks, Murano glass decorations, and miniature gondolas—typical Venetian souvenirs. Young musicians played their violins, and the voices of opera singers lifted up over the plaza. I again told Gary how overwhelming the beauty of this city was to me. I had to stop walking—the tears were streaming down my face as fast as I could wipe them away. Gary put his arm around my waist and assured me it was okay to cry.

What I did not say at the time was that I was overcome not only because of the beauty, but also because I once again had a feeling of having been here in a past life. I had visions of women wearing eighteenth-century gowns and men dressed in formal attire, all dancing the Viennese Waltz while wearing elaborate masks. It was a wonderful but unsettling experience because I couldn't understand where the visions were coming from. I later told Gary about this vision, but when he asked me more about it, I couldn't explain what I had seen or why.

The next morning, we went to the hotel restaurant, an intimate café that overlooked the Grand Canal. A salmon-colored linen tablecloth covered our table, and a red rose was placed in a vase at the center. A blue-and-white-striped canopy helped protect us from the morning sun, and the café was surrounded by greenery and colorful, fragrant flowers. The buffet breakfast presented a delicious array of fruits, pastries, organic jams and honey, cheese plates, and salmon. The weather was warm, but the sunshine and breeze from the ocean made for a perfect day. We watched the gondolas and water taxis pass back and forth across the canal, savoring our time together in this exciting environment.

After our breakfast, we returned to St. Mark's Square, where I was once again drawn to the masks, feeling a strong sense of passion and intrigue. As I looked at them, I felt I was looking for a part of myself. That afternoon I bought Gary a card with a mask on it to express the love I felt for him in this romantic city. I also sent a card with a mask on it to Gary's half sister, Pauline, because this trip reminded me of the mysterious connection we had when we first met.

I had met Pauline about a year prior in Ogden, Utah, along with Gary's stepmother, Helen. Gary did not know Pauline very well since she was older than him and they'd never lived in the same house. But when Pauline came out to greet us, she'd looked at me and said, "Don't I know you?"

"Not that I know of," I'd responded. "I've never been to Utah." Yet I'd felt like I had known her for years, and we connected immediately. Gary later told me that he had been perplexed as to what was going on between us; it certainly was a mystery to me as well. We maintained our relationship after this initial meeting by writing letters, and the mystery of the masks reminded me of the mystery of our connection.

I think part of my fascination with the masks was that they were works of art. Some represented classical gods and goddesses, and they came in all sorts of colors. Some masks had happy faces with designs that were sad and scary. And when I saw these masks, I saw a story behind them. I think each of us has a private mask we wear when we are alone and a separate mask we wear out in public. The mask we choose to wear depends upon who we are with and the circumstances—for instance, whether we're with a trusted friend or a stranger.

I also thought of my dear friend Suzanne. We had become close friends while attending a nursing program in Illinois and supported each other through both our nursing degrees and our divorces. And like my experience with Pauline, Suzanne and I had also had an instant personal connection. She loved Venice the most of all the many places she had traveled, and I wondered if my affinity for this place meant we all had been in this city together sometime in the far past. The depth of the feeling of having been here before was perplexing to me.

During this trip, I also was reminded of the importance of communication in a relationship. I tried to explain to Gary the importance of the masks and my emotional reaction to them, but it was difficult since I could not quite understand it myself. One day, as I was looking for a mask to buy as a symbolic gift for myself, I wanted Gary to be with me so I could talk with him about the masks and how I felt. However, once he saw me looking at the masks, he headed off to do his own thing. Later that evening, I told him that the masks had come to mean a lot to me, even though I could not adequately explain why, and that I wished he had been with me. Gary listened carefully and responded, "I had no idea that you felt so passionate about them, and I must admit, I don't fully understand what you are experiencing emotionally." This was a good lesson for me: we can't know how another person feels unless they tell us about it. So, I needed to be more specific in my communication with Gary if I wanted him to understand what was important to me and how I was feeling.

I was given an opportunity to apply this lesson the next day, when we went to a store that sold Murano glass. The store was very busy, and the sales staff were pressuring us to make a purchase. Gary wanted to find a piece to bring home, but I was tired and had no interest in buying anything in that moment. I just wanted to "be."

Gary noticed my demeanor and asked, "You don't want to shop or buy anything here?"

I felt bad because I knew he wanted to take his time and look around at all the interesting and beautiful glass pieces, and I instinctively wanted to brush off my feelings to suit his needs. However, I remembered the lesson I had learned, so I told him how overwhelmed I was feeling. He responded, "I understand, let's look at a few pieces to see if we can find something we like, and then we will go and get some lunch. What do you think?" I agreed, happy that we were both able to communicate our desires and needs.

That evening, we went for another walk in St. Mark's Square and enjoyed the music. The opera singing in the background was soothing to my soul, and I felt refreshed after a busy day. We sat down at a café and enjoyed a chicken sandwich and coffee as we watched the scenes unfold around us. And after our dinner, we happened to find the glass piece we were looking for: a chocolate-brown glass figurine of a couple holding each other, titled "The Lovers." It was the perfect symbolic representation of our love.

I also chose to buy a mask that had a feminine face and was half gold, half black. The eyes were slanted, and the full lips depicted a slight smile. I felt this mask was a good choice because it symbolized my own personality. There is one part of me that is very open and another that is very private, and I felt the two colors represented each of these sides. I still have the mask on my bedroom wall to this day—a reminder of the mysteries I encountered in this beautiful city.

Venice

Venice was the perfect end to our European tour. London and Poland had allowed me to explore my past; Rome and Florence had given us the opportunity to enjoy our present as a blended family. And Venice, while also rooted in the past, felt like a step toward our future together. We learned more about each other and about how to communicate better. We also deepened our love and found the perfect symbols to remind us of this trip for years to come. This trip was everything I could have hoped for and more, and I couldn't wait for us to go on more adventures together.

THIRTEEN

The Biltmore House

After being together for four years, Gary and I decided to buy a house. We were both in our fifties now and wanted a permanent home where we could grow old together. We each made a list of what we wanted so that we could prioritize what was important to us—Gary wanted to avoid a long commute while I wanted a house with some privacy, preferably in a wooded setting. Neither of us wanted a large home, but we wanted enough room that our children could comfortably visit us.

We presented our list to our realtor, and then we began looking at houses. Gary was busy with his law practice while I was primarily teaching psychiatric nursing three days a week, as well as working part-time at Gary's office. So, on my days off I would explore houses in Orinda, Lafayette, and Moraga, all of which were about twenty minutes from Gary's office. It soon became clear that finding the right place for us wasn't going to be an easy task. I ended up looking at one hundred homes over the course of eight months, becoming increasingly frustrated that so many weren't what we wanted. I had not passed the bar exam to date, which was frustrating for me, and had not yet given up on retaking it again at a future time. I wanted to find our home so I could focus on furthering my career and on our family travels.

Given our lack of success, we decided to expand our search. Gary recalled a former client of his, Scott Morris, who was a realtor in the Danville area, which was just outside of where we had been looking so far. We contacted him and decided to work with him to find our ideal home since he knew this area well. He was also the perfect person to work with because he was mild-mannered and didn't try to give us the hard sell, letting us take the lead but stepping in when he needed to.

After looking at a few homes, we found what we were looking for in Alamo, a boutique area situated in an enclave between Walnut Creek and Danville. The two-bedroom, three-thousand-square-foot home was located on a hillside surrounded by one hundred oak trees on an acre and a quarter of property. The gray and white house was set back from the one-way street, behind a white stucco half wall with red-brown bricks on top, which matched the brick trim along the curved driveway. There was a large attached two-car garage on the right of the house, and a turret window in the front added to the classic charm.

Gary and I looked at one another with anticipation as we followed Scott inside. We entered into a large, inviting great room that opened into the living room, dining room, and kitchen. The dining room held a large bay window that looked out over a flower garden that ran across the front of the house. The rooms were separated by floor-to-ceiling columns, and there was crown molding throughout the main floor. I was already in love.

We stepped into the sunken living room, which had beautiful Brazilian cherrywood floors, a raised dark brown marble fireplace surrounded by built-in oak bookcases, and two sets of French doors which led out to a redwood deck that ran the length of the house. The deck looked down upon several oak trees, and the property overlooked a golf course—though we were high enough and far enough away that we wouldn't have to worry about errant golf balls. Scott informed us that we may see all sorts of wildlife roaming the neighborhood: wild turkeys, deer, birds, squirrels, maybe even a coyote or bobcat if we were lucky. Gary loves birds, so this was a selling point for him.

As I looked around, I couldn't help but love the openness of the house and the privacy of the natural setting. The large properties in the area meant that there were hardly any neighbors nearby—an important feature for me. I grew up in a 1950s tract house with a small yard, where the neighbors were close to one another and would frequently gossip. I'd had enough of that environment as a kid; I enjoyed having a space all to myself. Plus, I love the woods, so the idea of being surrounded by trees was heavenly to me.

I returned my attention to the tour of the kitchen, which had three large windows looking out onto the trees on the side of the house, including two large California buckeyes. One of the most unique features of this home is that the kitchen did not look like a kitchen. The Sub-Zero refrigerator was discretely hidden by African wood cabinets, as was the microwave. The oven was hidden in a center island with a black countertop, and on the other side of the oven, there were wood shelves behind glass doors that you could place small family photos and decorations. The decor created a sense of warmth and comfort, and there was an easy flow of movement that would be perfect for large gatherings of family and friends. Off the kitchen was a laundry room, which also had plenty of storage.

Next, we went upstairs to see the large master bedroom, which had three alcoves each with a large window above a walnut bookshelf. We both could easily picture ourselves sleeping there. Just off the master bedroom was a cozy, custom-made library with white slanted walls, a built-in desk surrounded by bookshelves, and two windows that looked out over the front yard. Adjacent to this room was a large walk-in closet with custom-made drawers and a large window that overlooked the valley and deck. I immediately claimed this as my office and closet; Gary smiled and told me it suited me.

The final room was the master bath, which was located off a sitting room. There was a separate room behind a wood sliding door that had two sinks with oak cabinets underneath and a small window. Another door led to a room with a large walk-in tile shower and a forest-green tub with water jets. The toilet was in a separate room across from the shower. There were four windows above the tub that spanned the length of the bathroom so that no matter where you were in this room, you had a view of the valley and hills that stretched out toward San Francisco.

There was no question: we wanted this home. We put in an offer, and we were so happy when it was accepted—at least at first. Soon after, we found out that the couple who owned it were getting divorced, and the woman was forced to sell it even though she did not want to. As a result, I had mixed feelings when we went to sign the papers. I was happy for Gary and myself, but sad that our happiness was the result of her loss.

On November 10, 1994, Gary and I moved into our Biltmore

house. This was a turning point both in our relationship and in my personal life. I had not lived in a house since I'd divorced my ex-husband sixteen years ago. I had purchased and lived in a condo for seven years in the 1980s, but otherwise I'd been living in various apartments. This had worked well when I was single because it gave me the freedom to pursue school or career opportunities wherever they arose, but I had been longing to have a home and a sense of stability again—not only for myself, but also for Gary and me to share with our children.

Gary and I decided we were going to buy all new furniture for our house, only bringing with us the one sofa we'd bought together to place in the living room. We were starting from a clean slate in order to make our house into our home. That first year after moving in, we were busy shopping when we were not working, and we delighted in making these decisions together. We were fortunate that we liked the same type of furniture 90 percent of the time, which made this process much easier.

Now that we had enough space to accommodate everyone, we loved having the kids come and stay for a weekend or over the holidays. On our first Christmas Eve, the kids helped us in the kitchen as we cooked our first holiday meal together. I tried to make the experience easy and enjoyable by preparing most of the menu ahead of time—the corn chowder soup, cranberry dishes, and stuffing were all made in advance. Jen cut and mixed the green beans while Liz prepared the walnut salad. Lisa and Catherine prepared the warm bread and heated up the soup while Pat, who had arrived later, supervised. The five of them chatted about our trip to Rome and Florence the previous summer while they prepped the dishes—Lisa had not been able to join us on the trip, but she wanted to hear the stories.

Gary was responsible for carving the turkey while I took charge of the gravy. Finally, we all sat down together at our new dining room table, with the fireplace crackling in the background, and celebrated being together in our new home with a delicious dinner.

The Biltmore house would become the hub for many life experiences to come—love, loss, forgiveness, and choices we'd need to make during our golden years ahead. But for now, it was a place for our blended family to gather, connect, and grow closer together. And that was a dream come true.

FOURTEEN

Growing Together

While Gary and I were settling into our new home, I continued teaching psychiatric nursing at the VA hospital in Palo Alto as an adjunct faculty member with the University of San Francisco. I would get up at 4:30 a.m. three days a week to drive to the hospital and meet my twelve students for a preconference, in which we'd discuss any questions or concerns they had about the patients they'd been assigned for the day.

After entering the adult psychiatric unit, the students would look at their patients' charts to familiarize themselves with the person's diagnosis and behavior issues so they would know how to approach them. For instance, if a patient was depressed, the student would make sure the patient took their morning medication and would encourage them to get up out of bed and join the other patients for a community meeting. The patient did not have to talk if they did not want to, but it was beneficial for them to get up and dressed and out of their room for a short time. Their progress was measured by taking small steps each day, with the encouragement of the student or another staff member.

The students visited the unit throughout the semester and often got to see the patients make improvement in that time. In some cases, they would get to see a patient go home, though sometimes longer hospitalizations were required. Psychiatric nursing was usually one of the last clinical rotations the student experienced and the last course before graduation, and it was a great opportunity for them to learn about emotional care instead of just physical care. Sometimes, simply sitting with a patient for a short time and speaking with them was a healing process in itself. It was exciting to teach these young women and share in their professional journey.

During my time teaching this group of students, Gary decided to surprise me for my fifty-third birthday. While we were on our daily walk, he suggested that we take a different route than usual—a strange occurrence, as he had never made such a suggestion in our five years together. I was immediately suspicious. "Gary, what is going on? You are acting very strange."

"Nothing," he replied. "I just thought it would be fun to walk on this street." I agreed but told him he was acting weird.

Soon we came upon a house that I had never visited before. In front, I saw a black car with a big red bow on top—a brand new 1995 Mercedes C220 sedan. "Let's go up the driveway and look at it," he said.

"Gary, we don't know these people."

Laughing, he gestured for me to follow him. When I hesitated, he took my hand and pulled me up to see the card in the window, which read "Happy Birthday Lilly." He then reached into his shirt pocket and handed me the keys. A man and his wife emerged from the house with a big smile on their faces and a pair of scissors to cut the bow so I could drive it home. I soon learned that the man's name was Peter, and he was the person who sold the car to Gary.

I cried tears of joy and disbelief. I turned around and gave Gary a big hug and thanked him for the best birthday present I'd ever received, overwhelmed by my love for him.

As I opened the car door and sat down onto the soft tan leather seat, I breathed in the new car smell. I put my hands on the steering wheel so I could take it all in, and as I looked around the car, it finally started to sink in that it was mine. Gary got in the passenger seat, and I drove off with the biggest grin on my face. The car handled beautifully, and I could hardly wait to take the long drive to the hospital the next morning.

The next day, after my students were finished with their clinical work, they saw me get into my new car and gave me a thumbs up, shouting "Congratulations!" It was so sweet.

This gift will always be a memorable one for me. My parents never could have afforded such a gift, so I never expected something like this from them, or from anyone. I also couldn't believe the time and effort he had put in to surprising me with it. To me, this gift showed the depth of his love for me, and I will always be grateful for it.

May 1995 was a significant month for both Liz and Lisa—they were both graduating from college. Gary and I were glad that we were able to attend both ceremonies and be a part of this momentous occasion in their lives.

First, we went to New York to attend Liz's graduation from Adelphi University, in which she received her master's degree in social work. She looked so beautiful and happy in her black and gold gown as she confidently walked down the aisle to accept her diploma. She had worked hard to achieve her degree, working part-time during her two-year studies and living with her aunt Kat out on Long Island.

After the ceremony, the family all gathered around Liz to congratulate her. This was Gary's first time meeting my ex-husband, Ed, and his side of the family. Gary was introduced to Ed; his brother, Jerry, and his wife, Pat; their two daughters, Karen and Tara; and Ed's sister, Kat. I myself had not seen them in years, since they all lived in New Jersey and New York. Pat and I kept in touch for a while after Ed and I divorced—we had always gotten along well, especially since we were both nurses—and I visited the family several years earlier in New Jersey on my way to a nurses' convention. However, the distance made visiting difficult.

It was wonderful to see my two nieces, and we had a chance to chat and catch up on their lives. They were close in age to Liz, and I learned they were both in graduate school—Karen was working on her master's degree in occupational therapy, and Tara was in law school. We were all happy to be together to celebrate this significant event for Liz; she was beaming, and I was so proud of her.

After everything wrapped up, Gary and I went out to Massapequa Park to see my side of the family. They weren't able to attend the graduation ceremony since there were only so many seats available, but Liz was close with my family and saw them frequently during her studies.

Growing Together

My mother, age seventy-four, lived in the same house where I had been raised since I was eight years old; my dad had passed away from a sudden heart attack in 1982. She lived with my brother Guy and his girlfriend, Carol Ann. My brother Sonny and his wife, Joey, were also there when we visited, along with their daughter, Angela, who was a year younger than Liz.

Gary had met my family several times over the past five years because we would fly to New York to visit at least once a year. They loved Gary, and he enjoyed his time with them. We spent the afternoon hanging out together and catching up on our work, travels, and new home.

My relationship with my mother had not always been the best, which I wrote about in detail in my first memoir. At this time, though, my mother and I were finally healing our relationship. While we were visiting after Liz's graduation, Gary and I invited her to stay with us so we could share our new home with her, and she agreed to come out the following year. She'd always wanted to see San Francisco, and more importantly, she relished every chance to see her grandchildren, Pat and Liz, with whom she'd always been close.

A week later, we were on a train from New York City to Yonkers, New York, to attend Lisa's graduation from Sarah Lawrence College. Lisa also looked incredible in her black cap and gown as she walked to the podium to receive her diploma in art with confidence and grace. Gary and her mother, Liz, were especially proud of her, and so were the rest of her family.

We celebrated this special day with a dinner at a small Italian restaurant in New York City. Gary and I enjoyed being with Liz, Liz's brother, and Lisa's boyfriend. We had all met at a previous gathering, and it was enjoyable to see everyone and reconnect over a delicious dinner. Liz's brother was in the medical field in San Diego, and because of my nursing background, I always found our conversations to be easy and interesting. He and Liz were very close, and Gary always spoke highly of him.

Lisa and her boyfriend had been together a couple of years, and they looked forward to deciding where to live. Currently they were considering Boston, where he had family, or New York City, where Lisa thought she might be able to develop her career as an artist. The world was wide open to them as they began this new phase of their lives, and we were excited to see where the future would take them.

☼

Later that same summer, we had planned a two-week trip to London and Paris with my children, Pat P and Liz, as well as Gary's daughter Catherine and her boyfriend, Pat M. Gary and I decided to extend our trip and do a little traveling on our own ahead of time since the kids were busy with their work commitments.

We arrived at the Lucknam Park Hotel in Bath in late July. The decor of the mansion was very similar to the places we'd stayed the previous summer in London, with its cream walls and lovely red and gold tapestries. It was a place for us to unwind from our busy lives, find balance, and reconnect.

One of the interesting places we visited was the Roman Baths, which were built in AD 70. This was a place where Romans would clean themselves by putting oil on their skin and then removing it with a metal scraper called a strigil. The Roman Baths is one of the best preserved remains in the world, and it was interesting to see how the Romans lived at this time in history as well as one of the ways these people enjoyed spending time together.

Another fascinating place Gary wanted to share with me was Stonehenge, which he had visited on a previous trip. When we arrived, I was amazed at the sight of these massive stones surrounded by nothing but open countryside. It was built 4,500 years ago by a preindustrial farming society, and one theory is that they used tools made of bone and stone to create the blocks. I couldn't imagine how any human being could build the monument that stood before our eyes.

Experiences like this are why I love travel so much. Through visiting many different places in the world, we are invited to see and learn so much more about life and the capacity of human beings.

After our time in Bath, Gary and I headed to London to meet up with our family. We were all staying at the Radisson Blu Edwardian Berkshire Hotel, which was centrally located to Hyde Park and to some boutique shops on Bond Street. We thought this would be a good place for the kids to get over their jet lag while seeing some popular tourist sights.

Catherine and Pat M arrived early in the morning and wanted a chance to rest from their long flight from Seattle, Washington. When Pat P and Liz arrived, they were tired but excited to go on the red bus tour that visits the iconic sites in London. We sat on the upper deck, where we got a great view as we drove past sights like Trafalgar Square and Westminster Abbey. Gary and I had seen these landmarks on our previous trip, but we enjoyed watching and listening to their enthusiasm as they shouted out to each other, "Look, there is Big Ben! Hey, look over here, there is Buckingham Palace!" I gave Gary's arm a squeeze to express my happiness at being able to bring my two children on this wonderful trip. I know he felt the same about being able to spend more time with Catherine, especially since she had expressed feelings that her father was not there for her in her early years due to the contentious divorce from his first wife.

The next morning, after a delicious buffet breakfast, Pat P went to the London/Waterloo station to pick up his girlfriend, Ingrid, who would be joining us on the rest of our trip. They had been seeing each other for almost a year, and she was already in Europe to see her brother who was in Germany on vacation. We'd met Ingrid before on several occasions and liked her, so Gary and I invited her to join us. It would be a good opportunity to get to know her better.

One of the highlights that we shared together was seeing *Only the Lonely*, the story of the late Roy Orbison's life, at the Piccadilly Theatre. He'd been Gary's favorite singer, known for songs such as "Pretty Woman," "Crying," and of course, "Only the Lonely." Gary could not have been any happier to see this play, and we all enjoyed the music.

We made the most of our time in London. We visited Westminster Abbey, took a trip to Leeds Castle, and explored Trafalgar Square. We went to see *The Mousetrap* at St. Martin's Theatre as well as the English National Ballet's performance of *Romeo and Juliet*. The kids were clearly having a wonderful time; they would thank us during the day and individually expressed their gratitude to us. And at dinner one evening, Pat P spoke up on behalf of everyone and said, "We cannot thank you both enough for this awesome trip and the experiences that we have had with you." It was very heartwarming to know this trip was bringing them so much joy, and I'm so glad we could make it happen.

Gary and I could not leave London without sharing the magnificent Lanesborough Hotel with everyone. We all enjoyed their delicious buffet breakfast in the open-air dining room and talked about our favorite moments from the trip.

The next day, we all arrived at the London/Waterloo Station to take the underground train to Paris, where we would spend another week together. None of us had been there before, and I was particularly excited as I had always wanted to visit this romantic and artistic city.

Ingrid spoke French quite well, so we relied on her language skills on many occasions. She was an attractive young woman, with blue eyes and blond hair that fell softly around her face, and I enjoyed watching her communicate with the people around us. Her tone of voice was friendly, and her energetic disposition was revealed by her fast speech. Pat P was more reserved and deliberate, so the two of them complemented each other well. I loved watching them together as we explored this beautiful city. I also loved watching the three girls interact; Liz, Catherine, and Ingrid were all close in age, and we would often hear them chatting and laughing together.

We stayed at the Hôtel de l'Abbaye Saint-Germain, a former convent for Benedictine nuns. The decor was very colorful, with charming floral fabrics throughout the rooms. There was a garden with a glass roof, and we would eat our breakfast there in the morning before heading off to our activities for the day.

Paris did not disappoint. The ambience of the city was so European with its architecture and outdoor cafés. The Eiffel Tower was amazing, and the Louvre was breathtaking and overwhelming with all its artistic beauty. It was especially wonderful to actually see the Mona Lisa in person—there is nothing like walking into a museum and experiencing the true beauty of art. There was a sense of camaraderie among the children, who loved joking and telling stories around the dinner table each night. I savored every moment, feeling very fortunate that we could take this wonderful trip together and build these family connections.

As a symbol of our trip, Gary and I purchased a painting from a well-known French artist which hangs over our living room fireplace. The image depicts three boats with red and white sails entering a small harbor called Saint-Alban, a fifteenth-century city with two round brick towers on each side of the entrance, along with people walking along the shoreline. Whenever we look at this painting, it reminds us of our family trip, and reminds me of fulfilling my teenage dream to visit this incredible city.

FIFTEEN

The State of the World Forum

One of the most interesting weekends that Gary and I shared was when we participated in the first State of the World Forum.

This event was organized by Mikhail Gorbachev, the founder of an organization called the Gorbachev Foundation. Gorbachev was instrumental in helping end the cold war after the Berlin Wall came down in 1989. Now he wanted to bring together some of the most influential individuals in the world from eight specific groups—senior states people, current political leaders, business executives, scientists, artists, intellectuals, spiritual leaders, and youth—to create a working dialogue that would give birth to the first global civilization and generate solutions to critical global challenges. He called this group the State of the World Forum and planned for it to be held in San Francisco in September 1995.

Gary had been invited to participate in the Forum through a business contact, Jacqueline Neuwirth, the year prior. Gary told me then, "I made an early decision to accept the invitation, although doing so came at great financial expense. I felt from the beginning that this was an important experience for me in ways that I couldn't fully understand." As the event gathered momentum, Gary wanted me to be involved, so I signed up as well.

We met many important people who will be mentioned here, and it was an exhilarating and memorable time for me. Not only were we excited to be a part of this important forum, but it was also fun to have personal contact with these celebrities. I will highlight the most significant conversations and people that I remember meeting—interactions that have stuck with me to this day.

The events started on Wednesday September 27 with a VIP reception, which we were lucky enough to be invited to. We arrived at the Fairmont hotel and took the elevator up to the penthouse suite, where we met up with Jacqueline Neuwirth. We sipped cocktails in the elegant suite overlooking the Bay until Mikhail and Raisa Gorbachev arrived. They circulated around and met everyone, and we finally got a chance to shake Gorbachev's hand and have a few minutes to talk with him. He was a pleasant-looking man with a warm smile and a balding head with his signature birthmark. Gary told him that he felt lawyers were underrepresented at this conference; Mikhail laughed and reminded him that he was also a lawyer. Our impression was that he was very down-to-earth and not carried away by self-importance. I do not recall Mikhail using a translator for this meeting, even though he used one for his speech later on at the conference.

Other celebrities arrived including, to our surprise, Shirley MacLaine and Dennis Weaver. We got a chance to speak with her a little bit about her book, *Out on a Limb*, which had helped Gary quit drinking and launch his spiritual journey.

Then, toward the end of the reception, Ted Turner and Jane Fonda swept into the room. Turner was a rather loud, slap-you-on-the-back kind of fellow who certainly didn't take a back seat to anyone (including Gorbachev). He moved through the room, making sure that everybody got a chance to see him, but he didn't appear to connect with anyone. Time Warner had just taken over Turner's empire, and while we didn't notice any direct conversation about it, it was sure to be on everyone's minds.

Gary observed that Turner was the kind of guy who would stand up and start ad-libbing without putting much thought into what he was going to say. By the end of the night, we both came away with the impression that it was surprising a person like that could be the head of one of the most important companies in the world.

As we left the reception to head to the welcome dinner, Gary and I happened to walk out at about the same time as Turner and Fonda. Fonda looked at me and said, "Don't I know you from somewhere?"

I laughed and said, "Not in this life." We rode the elevator together and walked into the Grand Ballroom where dinner would be served. As we looked at the huge crowd that had already gathered, she confessed that she was feeling nervous. I suggested she take a deep breath, and she responded, "I know I should breathe, but I forget."

I felt surprisingly calm and nurturing toward her, I think because I sensed her vulnerability and saw her as a friend, not a famous person. The fact that she had asked if she knew me helped break the ice and made it easier for me to see her as a peer.

We were fortunate to be assigned to the table closest to the podium, right next to the table of Jane Fonda and Ted Turner. Carl Sagan was at our table with his wife, but since he was sitting across from us, we didn't get to talk with him. It was incredible to see all these celebrities here and know that they supported this organization and its goals. They added an additional legitimacy to the event and underlined the importance of what we were doing here.

Mayor Frank Jordan gave a warm and pleasant welcome to Mr. Gorbachev as well as the entire Forum audience. Ted Turner then introduced George Shultz, who offered personal reminiscences of his meetings with Mikhail Gorbachev when Shultz was Secretary of State between 1982 and 1989. He talked a lot about how he reported to President Reagan that Gorbachev was "really a different kind of leader" than they'd ever dealt with before. His remarks were pleasant, personal, and very well-received.

Gorbachev then took the stage to a very warm and prolonged standing ovation. His remarks throughout the speech were marred somewhat by the translation from Russian to English—he and the interpreter would occasionally overlap and step on each other's toes. Regardless, Gorbachev was able to give us a clear vision of what he hoped to accomplish at this forum. It was a real privilege to sit there, just a few feet from the podium, and watch this historic event unfolding before our eyes. Gary and I came away from this experience with the sense of having been a part of something important, and we were full of enthusiasm for the days ahead.

The next day, we arrived just after the opening of the plenary session by Mikhail Gorbachev with a brief introduction from Jim Garrison, a former district attorney, and his co-chair Thabo Mbeki, the vice president of South Africa and the heir apparent to Nelson Mandela. Then Carl Sagan and Zbigniew Brzezinski each gave a twenty- to thirty-minute speech on where we were headed in the twenty-first century. Carl Sagan talked about the new and ongoing research into finding new galaxies and searching for other life forms. As part of this, he showed some amazing slides that included pictures from space. The last shot, which was taken from Voyager Two, showed a picture of Earth from the furthest spot out in space. It was framed by pictures of six other planets, and Earth appeared to be a small pale blue dot in a ray of sunshine. This picture formed the basis of his new book at the time, called *Pale Blue Dot*. Although Gary considered Sagan to be way too scientifically grounded and not in touch with anything metaphysical, an aspect of life that Gary felt was important to consider, we both enjoyed his remarks.

Brzezinski, who had been the security adviser for Jimmy Carter and was now a college professor, gave a hard-hitting speech on the great decline in our values throughout the past century. He was particularly upset about television violence. He claimed that the twentieth century was by far the worst in the history of humanity due to the terrible killings by the Nazi and Stalin regimes as well as the eighty million people who had apparently been killed by their governments. His outlook was rather gloomy, although his delivery was passionate.

We sat with Mr. Brzezinski during lunch, and our conversation with him was inspiring. Gary was a bit more optimistic about the future of humanity, so he and Brzezinski ended up having a very spirited discussion. Brzezinski said that his son-in-law was an attorney, and that the two of them frequently argued. I could understand why—although Brzezinski was friendly, he was also quite strongly opinionated. He reminded me of my Polish grandparents, and I chatted with him about our shared Polish heritage.

After lunch, we had our first roundtable session. These sessions consisted of twenty people engaging in short discussions—the presenters had five minutes to talk on a specific subject, and then everyone else at the table got two to three minutes to share their own thoughts. I chose a session on leadership called "The Paradox of Success" while Gary went to one called "The Global Crisis of Spirit and the Search for Meaning: Asian and Western Perspectives on Crisis and Meaning." I think we all came away from these talks having learned something. The one I attended was very intense, and it took me a while to digest all the information I was given.

Following these discussions, we attended a reception in the Terrace Room. Here we met and spoke with several people, including Dr. Matthew Fox, a well-known excommunicated Catholic priest and spiritual leader from Oakland. He was a nationally known author and speaker, and he appeared to be a wonderfully humble and humorous man.

The dinner that night was opened by poet and author David Whyte, who read a poem before each dinner and lunch. He was eloquent in his readings and added a good deal to the ambience of all our evenings. After Whyte finished, Deepak Chopra gave a keynote speech that was, in essence, about making the world a better place.

That evening, Gary and I ended up sitting next to Shirley MacLaine and having another chance to speak with her. We talked to her about her books and discussed our relationship at length, and she listened attentively to our stories. These discussions made me appreciate my life with Gary and recognize how much I had changed in the past five years, going from being a single woman to being in a committed relationship. With this recognition came the acknowledgment that I was a much happier person today because I had found the man I loved and wanted to spend my life with. Talking with Shirley reminded me of the frustrations of the dating world. I had enjoyed being single and focusing on my career, but my life was enhanced with Gary through the richness of our love and the blending of our families.

At the end of the dinner, Shirley gave us her address and phone number. A few weeks later, she sent us copies of all her books, which were personally signed with a lovely note from her saying how she enjoyed spending time with us and hearing our relationship story.

On Friday September 29, Gary and I chose to attend a Forum dialogue called "Expanding the Boundaries of Humanness." The discussion was moderated by Alan Jones, the rector of the Grace Cathedral, and involved several panelists. Perhaps the crowning moment of the session came when Thich Nhat Hanh, a Vietnamese Buddhist monk who was taking part in the discussion, entered the room. As soon as he entered, everyone became completely riveted by him. He was a small, unassuming man, yet his presence was over-powering. He spoke about his Buddhist tradition and how he would look at a flower and see in it the sunlight that had helped it grow. As he got further into feeling what was in the flower, he began to see all parts of it, including the clouds, the rain, the earth, and eventually, himself. He spoke about ultimately emerging with the flower in his own experience, which to me represented how all human beings are connected to and part of the universe.

On the last day of the Forum, we were treated to a powerful speech by Jane Goodall. After working with chimpanzees for thir-ty-five years, she noted the incredible similarities between humans and chimpanzees. I was surprised to learn we share 99.9 percent of our genes, and that chimpanzees are able to experience emotions such as grief, loss, pain, and love. This knowledge may shift our belief that we're the most evolved species on our planet, let alone the universe. We didn't get to meet her personally, but she inspired us to learn more about her work.

Overall, the State of the World Forum offered us experiences that neither of us will ever forget. Everyone, famous or not, got involved in discussions with one another, and each person had something to add to the conversation. We felt we were indeed part of forming a new way of thinking, and I felt that the ripple effect from all these people going out into their various communities would be profound. As for us, we had a life-changing experience that would likely affect us in ways we couldn't begin to understand yet. That's the fun of life—you can never quite know exactly where each new experience will take you.

In retrospect, yes, the Forum made an ongoing impact on our lives by giving us the sense that we could help make the world a better place. My family and I are so very sad to be leaving our current global legacy to our children and our grandchildren; this is not the world that we envisioned when Gary and I joined the State of the World Forum. Hopefully we will start to see some positive change soon. In the meantime, all we can do is try to make a difference on our own personal level. After all, even small improvements can lead to big changes over time.

SIXTEEN

Africa

In 1996, Gary and I decided to make a trip to Africa. This continent had been fascinating and mysterious to me ever since the Mau Mau uprising, which occurred when I was a teenager. The uprising began in 1952 as a reaction to inequalities and injustices in British-controlled Kenya and lasted until 1960. The colonial administration responded by cracking down on the rebels, resulting in many deaths. I remember being curious about who these people were and where they lived, and that curiosity had only grown over the years. Gary had been to Africa several years earlier, and he was excited to share this country with me.

Finally, the day arrived. As the plane lifted up and took us off into the sunset, Gary and I looked into each other's eyes, held hands, and sighed a big breath of relief that we were finally beginning our month-long vacation.

After landing in London for an extended layover, we checked in at the Lanesborough Hotel and then relaxed by getting a massage and taking a walk along the Thames River. We also spent time just being together, watching *Richard III* while eating in our room or going out for dinner at the Spaghetti House, our favorite restaurant. After two days, we felt refreshed and ready for Africa and the adventures that awaited us there.

We arrived in Nairobi's Jomo Kenyatta International Airport at 9 a.m. and were met by Mike Rainey, our host, who took us to Serata Suruwa for a two-night stay. Serata Suruwa was a wildlife estate located ninety kilometers south of Nairobi and owned by Michael and Judith Rainey, American naturalists who had made the open spaces of Kenya their home. We got to our camp about midday and were pleased to see that our tent had a comfortable double bed, a separate toilet, and a "shower"—or rather, a suspended bucket filled with hot water. We were out in the middle of nowhere, with open hills all around us and blue sky as far as our eyes could see. I was not a camper, so this was definitely out of my comfort zone, but this seemed like the natural place to stay in a country where the natives lived in mud huts and walk miles for their food and water.

Two other couples joined us for an excellent lunch in the veranda tent, and we all went for a two-hour walk up the bluff to where we could see some animals several hundred yards below—giraffes, elands, and a few zebras. The view of the grasslands and the wildlife was an exhilarating contrast to the world we'd left behind in the States.

That night and the next we had excellent hot meals—fresh bread, steamed rice, fresh vegetables, and a green salad. Lunches were also hot with mashed potatoes, Swiss steak, vegetables, and fresh baked dessert. The breakfasts included omelets, sausage, fresh toast, muffins, hot cakes, and juice, all made without electricity. The staff were pleasant but did not look at us or talk directly to us, and they would bow slightly as we passed by them to sit at the table. After they prepared the meals and placed them on a side table, buffet style, they stood along the side of the room while we had our dinner and removed the dishes as soon as we finished. There appeared to be an unspoken rule that we should not engage in any conversation with the staff outside of the guides assigned to us for the walks and animal explorations. I did not think much about it at the time, just simply accepted it as part of their culture.

The following day we took a three-and-a-half-hour walk along the top of the hill with Mike and two guides. Mike was an interesting man. He was a British biologist in his sixties who had decided to give up his life in London and come to Africa to find meaning and purpose in his life. He must have found it, because he'd stayed there ever since, working to conserve the land and have farmers live with the wild animals.

For the next leg of our trip, we flew from Nairobi to Nanyuki and were then transported to the wilderness trails located on the Lewa Downs ranch. This was the home of the Craig family, who have managed this 50,000+ acre ranch for over three generations. It was the home of Africa's most successful rhinoceros sanctuaries, and since Gary had a fondness for rhinos, he was especially happy to be here.

At this ranch we stayed in a more comfortable luxury thatched cottage, and the property had horses and giraffes roaming about. It was easy to forget about the wildlife, so as we walked back to our cottage in the dark after dinner on our first evening, Gary and I walked right into a giraffe! We had a good laugh about it when we got back to our room—it's not the kind of situation you ever imagine finding yourself in.

One of my favorite experiences at this camp was getting up early and going out on horseback with Gary and two guides to see the animals up close. I had always loved horses, but I was also afraid of them because they are so strong. I took horseback riding lessons in my fifties and enjoyed them for a while, but the lessons became more challenging, and I eventually stopped because I was afraid of falling and breaking a bone. So, I went on this morning ride with a bit of trepidation, but I felt the need to overcome my fear so that it wouldn't take away from this special experience. I had previously read the book *Feel the Fear and Do It Anyway* by Susan Jeffers, Ph.D., and I decided to use this title as my motivation to move forward. I felt safe with the guides and with Gary riding behind me, so I took some deep breaths and made the decision to enjoy this ride.

I'm so glad I was able to move past my fear and fully take part in this experience. The animals didn't see us as a threat while we were on horseback, so we were able to get closer than I ever thought possible. Our group was able to get fifteen feet from a giraffe, and we got close enough to a group of zebras that I could have touched them with my hand. It all seemed both natural and surreal, and we really felt like we were in Africa!

The staff then set up a surprise breakfast in the bush that included coffee, hot chocolate, oatmeal, eggs, sausage, baked bread, and muffins. Gary and I put our arms around each other as we took in the open countryside and gave thanks for being in this incredible country.

The area was abundant with wildlife, so we went out on open Land Cruisers for several hours each day to get a glimpse of the many animals. We saw impalas, zebras, waterbucks, giraffes, and monkeys up close as well as some baboons off in the distance. But for Gary, getting within thirty feet of some rhinos—two males and one female—and hearing the crunching noises as they ate the grass was pure heaven. One day, as dusk approached, we saw something exciting through our binoculars: a leopard eating its prey in the center branch of a large tree. It was a bit too far away and a bit too dark to get a photograph, but it was still a sight we shall never forget.

Gary and I became more and more relaxed on the trip as we awakened each day to a new adventure at our camp. The veranda at our lovely cottage was the perfect place to take in the fresh air and listen to the birds chirping around us. I believe this time away to just be with each other was important for our relationship and helped us realize what we meant to one another. We had traveled together before, and Gary and I often expressed our love for one another, but this experience felt much more intimate. Without the hustle and bustle of activities to do and sights to see, we were able to just relax and enjoy one another. And as a result, I felt emotionally closer to him than I ever had before.

The relaxing nature of our trip benefited us physically as well. Gary said he felt rested and didn't have the usual neck and back aches that had bothered him for a while. "I am feeling 100 percent," he said one morning as he got up to stretch, then we hugged each other before heading off on another horseback adventure.

The weather this day was great—warm but not hot with a pleasant breeze. We saw a two-month-old zebra nursing from her mother, and then later we saw two male zebras get into a sudden and violent fight. I was a bit nervous about how we would be affected by the fight since it happened not far from where we were riding on our horses; thankfully, we weren't impacted, and the zebras did not appear to be badly hurt.

We came back for breakfast and then went back out for a three-hour game run in an open Land Cruiser. Gary got to see three rare black rhinos, which watched warily as our safari Cruisers passed. We learned that the prevalence of poachers was one of the reasons for them being so cautious.

One evening, instead of going out for a game drive, we spent some time at the home of David and Delia Craig, who owned the ranch. They were in their seventies, and we enjoyed talking about the world in these fast-moving times over cocktails. After that, we simply relaxed in our room and enjoyed our time together. Gary was reading *Emotional Intelligence* by Daniel Goleman and shared some of the insights with me by reading parts of a chapter on arguments and differences. In essence, it affirmed for us that talking with each other about what is bothering or upsetting us rather than holding it in and allowing it to fester was crucial to having a successful relationship.

Gary and I were not having any ongoing arguments or differences at this point in our relationship, but we both liked to read about relationship issues in order to keep improving ourselves. This book was of interest to both of us, and after reading a chapter or two, we would discuss what we each thought about the lessons within. This process helped us to discuss our personal viewpoints on the subject matter, learn about each other's feelings and concerns, and understand how any potential issues could be resolved.

One example would be our discussions around the subject of marriage. Both of us were quite satisfied with our decision not to get married, but I had some insecurities during our early relationship that would surface on occasion. So, we would share our thoughts about the pros and cons of getting married, to make sure both our needs were being met. We found it was better and healthier to have these important discussions at a time when we felt calm rather than angry, tired, or pressured by work stress, and this trip offered just the right environment for us to talk about these matters.

※

Our next stop was Ol Malo, "the place of the greater kudu." It was a five-thousand-acre ranch in Kenya owned by Colin and Rocky Francombe. Since Gary and I were one of two couples staying on the ranch at the time, we were offered an exclusive personal experience in this peaceful wilderness.

Our cottage was discreetly nestled on a cliff overlooking a watering hole frequented by giraffes. Past the watering hole was miles of rugged bush, with Mt. Kenya looming beyond. There was a total of three double guest houses, each with an ensuite bathroom and a private veranda surrounded by gardens of indigenous plants and green lawns. No matter what room we were in, we could see rugged hillsides and open land that stretched for miles and miles.

One of the selling features of this camp was a secluded infinity pool that overlooked the expansive face of Africa. Gary and I aren't especially interested in pools, but we absolutely had to experience this one. It was relaxing to be the only couple in the pool, and to be able to sit by the poolside with our arms around one another as we looked out at the magnificent view.

The next morning, a young Samburu man guided us along a nearby river and showed us various plants that could be used as a toothbrush, as skin care, and for medicinal purposes. We learned that the river was unsafe because a crocodile had recently eaten several goats that got too close to the banks. We also heard there were hippos nearby—one of the most dangerous creatures in Africa—though we did not see them. So, we made sure to keep out of the water.

The rest of the day was rainy, so Gary and I had a chance to rest and relax in our room after dinner. Life seemed so simple, and I loved that we were able to be together without our usual busy life schedules. In retrospect, this trip brought to our awareness how stressful our life had become in the past two years.

Another evening, we shared dinner with the other two couples and had a very philosophical discussion. It was a lively and interesting conversation, and since the others expressed interest in my opinions and life experiences, I felt free to express myself with ease. Gary was surprised at how verbal I was; he had not seen this part of me in our six years together. It is not that I felt I needed to keep anything from Gary, but rather that I had a tendency to hold back if the time was not right to discuss my feelings about a certain situation. At home, I was so wrapped up in work and family obligations that I didn't really allow myself to just be, and as a result I wouldn't always fully participate in the conversations around me. Here, we were relaxed and felt very comfortable and open with ourselves, so I was able to open myself up to these strangers and more fully discuss my views. I think this is the beauty of taking vacations—we can refresh ourselves and keep the love alive by seeing one another in a new way.

The next afternoon we went to the Samburu tribe settlements, called *manyattas*. We learned that traditionally, the Samburu men looked after the livestock—cows, goats, sheep, and camels—and were responsible for the safety of the tribe while the women were responsible for gathering vegetables and roots, caring for the children, and collecting water. We learned from our guide that the Samburu were a gerontocracy, which meant the elders ruled the tribe and decided when ceremonies such as weddings and circumcisions would occur.

I found it very illuminating to learn about the Samburu traditions around circumcision and how they were intertwined with the tribe's way of life. Entry into both womanhood and manhood is marked with a circumcision ceremony, and men and women are only able to get married once they are circumcised. The way they explained their point of view made the practice seem so natural, and yet it also seems so barbaric to my Western sensibilities. It was all a matter of perspective, which I think is an important lesson to be learned from traveling and experiencing other cultures and their beliefs.

We were invited into a mud-dung house owned by one of the Samburu families in the village. The building was made of mud, sticks, grass, cow dung, and cow urine, the combination of which repelled mosquitoes and kept the dwellers cool. Inside we were overcome with the smell of smoke from a fire burning, and we saw the blood and milk gourds lying in the corner of the room. The blood is obtained by precisely nicking the jugular artery of a cow, allowing the person to collect some blood without killing the animal. This blood is then mixed with milk and used as a ritual drink in special ceremonies for the sick. There was also a place in the house for the family's goat, which is a sacred animal to the tribe.

As we explored the village, we also noted a blacksmith making spears. Africans began extracting iron ore from the continent's rich deposits roughly 2,500 years ago, and blacksmithing had since become a widespread practice across sub-Saharan Africa.

Gary and I were privileged to see a Samburu dance at the invitation of our hosts, Colin and Rocky, who were known to the Samburu chief. Dancing is a significant part of their culture, serving as an important ritual. The dancers, who were all men, wore the traditional dress of the tribe: a striking red cloth wrapped like a skirt, a white sash, and many colorful beaded earrings, bracelets, anklets, and necklaces. Each piece of jewelry represented the status of the wearer; the more the person wore, the higher their rank within the tribe. For the ritual, the men danced in a circle and jumped high from a standing position.

This experience gave us a real sense of how the Samburu lived their lives every day. We also got to see how they interacted with the ranch owners and with the wildlife. It was a very enlightening experience that brough a completely different way of life into my awareness.

On another day, we took a camel ride through the African countryside, which I quite enjoyed. I'd had the opportunity to ride a camel during a previous trip to Egypt, but I'd decided not to take part because the camels were dirty and smelled awful. I had often wished I went on that camel ride, and now here was my chance to make up for that lost opportunity. Thankfully, these camels were clean and well taken care of, and the seat I was sitting on was colorful and comfortable. Gary also rode on a separate camel, but he was not as enthused as he didn't find his seat as comfortable. We did not see much game during this ride, but we did see the relatively rare oryx, which is a type of antelope with long, straight horns.

Africa

After breakfast, we boarded a private charter flight to Nanyuki to then catch Air Kenya's flight to Masai Mara, Kenya's most famous game reserve. We were staying at Rekero Camp, which was the home of Ron and Pauline Beaton and their oldest son, Gerard. Ron is known throughout East Africa as a talented game scout and one of Kenya's finest safari guides. The accommodations were described as "cozy, rustic cottages" near a waterhole often populated with elephants, baboons, buffalo, and the occasional lion.

When we arrived, we changed our "rustic cottage" for one of the units with a double bed. There was a nice watering hole in front of the cottage, populated by a few baboons and bushbuck when we arrived. However, the spiders in the cottage and the slug on the shower pipe did not make for my idea of a fun place to stay! I had flashbacks to our disappointing accommodations in Hana. At first, I would not go in, but since we had booked four days here I needed to overcome my fears once again. Gary was supportive, listening to me and once again applying logic to appease my fears. It worked.

Once I got over my fears, I did come to enjoy the camp. The sunsets were beautiful, and the game drives were interesting. We saw a number of wildebeests, a hyena, some elephants, a big bull buffalo, and some zebras. We also got to see a mother cheetah and her three cubs. It was great fun.

As we experienced each private home and camp, which had all been suggested by our travel agent, I learned that each one had their own particular personality. Each place we stayed offered a very special experience to learn from, and we came away from each experience having learned more about Africa than we would have by staying at the same resort for several weeks.

Our next stop was the famous Tarangire National Park, which is a favored retreat for experiencing vast wildlife. The camp here also allowed for night drives and guided treks through the bush, and it offered twenty luxury tents with private facilities to enjoy the privacy of Africa.

The highlight of being in this camp was seeing our first lions. We were out with a guide in a Land Cruiser which was fitted with roomy roof hatches so that you could stand up to use your camera or binoculars, and one walked right in front of us on the road. We then noticed a wildebeest carcass in a burned area off the road—sometimes the ranchers start grass fires to prepare the soil for crops—with three lions feasting on the kill. We were very excited to finally see them in the wild. Our guide told us that the restless zebras, wildebeests, and gazelles we had seen were on guard against the hungry cats.

As we made our way back, we encountered a problem. Just outside the camp, we noticed a big elephant about two hundred yards ahead of us who did not want us to pass. He trumpeted and flapped his ears, looking like he would charge at our vehicle. My heart pounded. I didn't like this situation one bit; this elephant could crash through acacia trees as if they were sticks of kindling. Finally, he walked backward and moved in another direction. The guide said that teenage males like this one will often act out and test their strength, but they will not charge the vehicles unless provoked. Regardless, I was relieved when we got back safe and sound. We wanted memorable, authentic experiences of Africa, and we certainly got one!

That evening. we enjoyed a big fire and took in the beautiful starry sky. We got to see Jupiter, the Scorpio constellation, and the Milky Way through the camp owner's telescope. We also enjoyed a delicious dinner with an Italian couple who were there for only one night. Unfortunately, Gary and I did not sleep well that first night; we were kept awake by the sound of what we believed was some poor animal being killed by a predator.

The next afternoon, we went on a long safari drive to find the big five—lions, leopards, rhinos, elephants, and African buffalo. I didn't think we'd see any more lions, but then we came across a roadside scene for our memory book. A pride of sixteen lions were lounging around two parked safari rigs, yawning, dozing, and seeking cover from the blazing midday sun. It was a heart-pounding encounter for Gary and me, though our guide was unfazed—after all, the whole idea of safari drives for any guest is to see as many of the big five animals as possible.

"The lions are just being lazy," he said. "They like the shade."

We watched them for a while, and we even saw the lead female hunt some zebras, though she did not charge. Still, it was an experience I'll never forget.

Soon we were off on a bumpy and dusty drive to our final destination, Sopa Lodge in Lake Manyara National Park, which was known for its variety of animal sights. It was worth the drive. We came upon lush forests with monkeys and elephants right by the road, just ten to fifteen feet from us. The monkeys were running all around us, and I worried that they might try and jump into our vehicle. I was also worried that the elephants might charge us, given our previous experience; thankfully, they ignored us as we drove by. Later, we saw twenty hippos half-submerged like fat logs in a cool-water pond, with more hippos standing out of the water. We were within twenty-five to thirty feet of some of them.

We then came across a huge baboon troop. Our guide told us that a troop could contain anywhere from dozens to hundreds of members that would groom and protect each other. As he was talking, we noticed the young baboons were playing together. Some camera-shy warthogs, armed with wicked tusks, waddled close to us, and there were many wildebeests near a lake in the distance.

On our first night at the lodge, Gary woke up at 2:45 a.m. due to some noise. Lo and behold, three huge Cape buffalo stood on the grass directly in front of our window, no more than ten feet away. Gary got the flashlight and awakened me, and we were both awestruck by these huge animals standing so close to us. We were also glad to be seeing them from the safety of our room.

Africa will remain a special place for us. It was a place of paradoxes; there was a sense of openness, simplicity, freedom, and adventure, and yet there was an underlying threat of the power of the wild animals around you. The guides and ranch owners who lived there carried rifles to protect both their property and their lives. Getting closer to nature like this allowed Gary and I to become closer with each other, and our love seemed to grow stronger with each new experience. I will always have fond memories of this trip, and of the time we got to spend together.

Africa

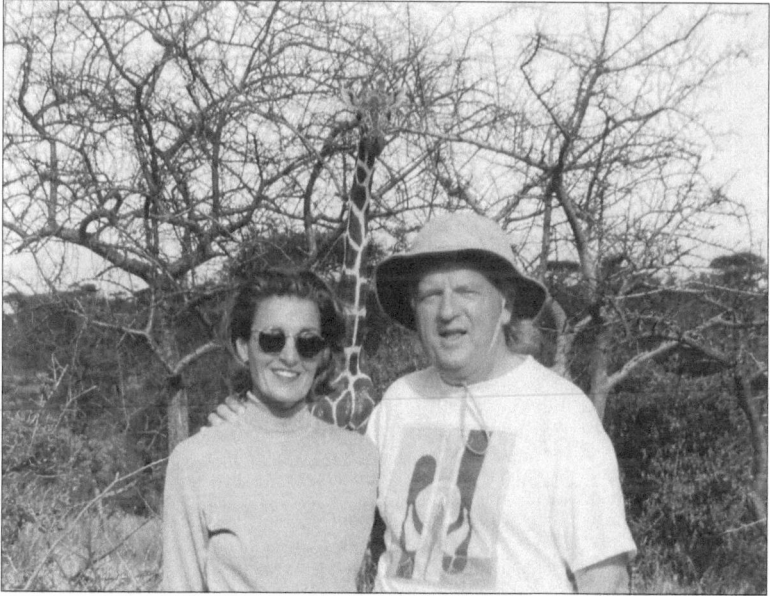

Lilly and Gary's first Africa trip, 1996

SEVENTEEN

Why Get Married? Why Not?

When Gary and I first started dating, we decided that neither of us was ready to get married. He had been divorced twice already and felt that marriage would destroy the wonderful relationship we had together; being divorced myself, I also didn't see the need to take that step. However, after three years of living together and learning each other's quirks and habits, Gary and I decided we were committed to each other and wanted to show this commitment to our kids, family, and friends. We had a small gathering in our apartment during the Christmas holidays, and that was that. Or so we thought.

After our fifth year together as a couple, Gary and I decided that while we still didn't see a need to get married, we wanted to have a larger ceremony to formalize our commitment to one another in the presence of our friends and family. The day we decided to do this, Gary said, "Wouldn't it be fun to have our ceremony at the exact time and day that we met five years ago?"

"What a romantic idea," I replied. I hugged and kissed him, glad to have a partner as romantic as I was.

Our first date was on the Saturday after Thanksgiving at 5:00 p.m., and this year we would be in Maui during that time for a California Trial Lawyers Association conference. We thought this would be the perfect time and place to celebrate our relationship, especially since many of our friends would be attending the conference.

When we began looking for a place to hold the ceremony, our top contender was the Wailea Seaside Chapel. Gary and I had seen this chapel several times on our beach walks over the years; it was our favorite walk in the world because of the stunning view of the blue-green ocean and the three small islands in the distance. The chapel was surrounded by a tranquil pond filled with brightly colored koi that seemed to beckon us to step into the building. When we had sat in one of the mahogany pews on a past vacation, I enjoyed an immediate sense of peace. Gary and I imagined our family and close friends sitting in this chapel with its raised altar surrounded by stained glass murals lit by the Maui sunset, and we decided this would be the perfect place to hold our ceremony. We couldn't wait to tell our kids about our plans, and when we did, they all expressed how excited they were to visit Maui and enjoy the Thanksgiving holiday together.

On November 25, 1995, the weather was sunny with a cool breeze, and we knew we'd enjoy the beautiful sunset we'd envisioned. The chapel was filled with our five children and their significant others, Gary's law partners and their families, and some of our closest friends. I wore a white silk Hawaiian dress with white sandals and a headpiece with white and pink flowers; Gary wore a blue shirt and sport jacket with tan pants. At the beginning of the ceremony, he placed a white lei around my neck, and I placed long green leis with many small leaves around his. We read a poem to each other, then expressed our vow to love and honor the other and not take each other for granted.

Next, we exchanged our gifts. I gave Gary an African warrior made of green verdite with black ebony stone. Gary had seen this art piece in a store window as we were exploring the island and had told me how much he liked this sculpture. I decided it would be a great gift, and a symbolic representation of both our connection to Maui and our relationship.

Gary surprised me by saying, "Lilly, will you please take my hand?" He placed a diamond ring on my finger and said, "This ring belonged to my mother, and it was given to me before she died. I want you to have it as a symbol of my love for you." I felt overcome with love for Gary as I knew he was very close to his mother.

At the end of the ceremony, we invited our guests to speak. Several guests offered very heartwarming words, but my favorite moment was when my twenty-eight-year-old daughter, Liz, shared how she felt. "Gary, you have made my mom so happy." She became close to tears and nodded to Gary's daughters. "I've loved our trips and time together. I love you guys!" I knew that they loved Liz as well. I felt close to tears myself upon listening to our family and friends share their happiness for us. It was so rewarding and heartwarming to see that our efforts to create a happy blended family were paying off.

After the ceremony, we then walked across the lovely lush tropical grounds of the Grand Wailea Resort to the Humuhumunukunukuāpua'a restaurant, which is named after one of the most widely recognized Hawaiian fish. To get to the entrance, we had to walk down a wooden bridge walkway that was floating on its own lagoon. As we did, I felt like I was floating on air, filled with love for Gary, our children, and our friends. Gary was walking close to me and put his arms around my waist, frequently expressing how happy he was and how much he was enjoying our special day.

The restaurant was made up of circular rooms with thatched roofs that were open on the sides, surrounded by tiki torches and tropical plants with the soft sound of waves in the background. After dinner, we walked along the ocean, holding hands and letting the waves rush over our bare feet as we looked back on our day and appreciated how much our relationship had grown over the years.

Gary and I were confident in our decision not to get married, but it wasn't a common or well-understood choice. Throughout our relationship, people would often ask us, "Are you married?" When we said no, the question became, "Are you planning to?" At first, these questions didn't faze me at all; I would just laugh and say we were happy as we were. Gary and I were both clear that we were just enjoying each other, and that time would tell where our relationship would go.

As the years went on, though, the questions began to bother me more and more. We were surrounded by married couples, making us the odd couple out among our lawyer friends. Even after our commitment ceremonies, I began to wonder what was wrong with me. Why didn't Gary want to marry me? Was our relationship not as strong as I thought it was? I talked with Gary about my feelings, and through these discussions I came to realize that while I was fine in my mind and heart to simply be committed to one another, the relentless questions were making me uncertain about the status of our relationship. I tried my best to shake these feelings, but they were persistent.

Shortly after our travels through Africa, I was in the living room putting away photos from our trip when Gary said, "Lilly, do you want to get married?" It turned out the questions had been bothering him as well.

Surprised, I answered, "Yes." My response came naturally and without hesitation, and we both stopped what we were doing to embrace.

After a second, I pulled back to look into his serious blue eyes. "Are you sure?"

"Yes, more than I ever thought possible," he said, embracing me even harder. "We've spent so many years defending why we did not want to get married. Let's change that to 'why not get married'!"

I thought about our kids', families', and friend's reactions to our news. I thought they would be happy for us, but that they also would likely wonder why it took us so long to take the leap.

Gary was eager to plan this special event. "What do you think about getting married on my sixtieth birthday next May? The more I think about, the more perfect it seems. Then I can't forget it or confuse it with my other two anniversaries." We both laughed, and I agreed that this was a great idea.

We called our kids to share the news, and of course they gave us hearty congratulations, as did our family and friends. I couldn't wait for us to get married, and to share this special day with our loved ones.

❋

Our wedding took place on May 18, 1997, seven years after we met. The day was beautiful and sunny, though a bit hot at 105°F. The plan was that we were all going to get ready together at our Biltmore house, and then we would head to a church in Lafayette for the service followed by a cocktail reception and dinner at the Roundhill Country Club.

While there were many parts of the day that I was looking forward to, I was especially eager to wear my wedding dress, designed by Badgley Mischka. I'd been going through all the wedding dress magazines for months when I came upon a dress that was worn by actress Julia Ormond at the recent Golden Globe Awards. As soon as I saw it, I knew that this was the dress I wanted to wear. I then met up with my childhood friend Sharon in New York so she could help me choose a wedding dress, and we headed straight to Saks Fifth Avenue. To my delight, the dress that I wanted was there, and in my size as well! I had to hold back my desire to scream with excitement.

The magazine had shown the simple, floor-length dress to be made of a soft, elegant lace with a matching jacket. However, the dress that I tried on was made of a heavy beaded material. Thankfully, the saleswoman said I could have it made without the beading, and my dress arrived in time for me to have a final fitting before the wedding day.

The morning of the wedding, our house was full of bridesmaids and groomsmen getting ready and posing for photographs. My wedding party included my daughter Liz as my maid of honor, with Catherine, Jen, Ingrid, and Gary's law partners' daughters, Bess and

Jaime, as my bridesmaids. On the groom's side was Gary's college friend Monte Ross as the best man, with my son Pat and Gary's law partners as the groomsmen. We all enjoyed a catered buffet breakfast as we got ready for the big day ahead.

The girls started early, getting their hair and makeup done in our kitchen in front of the large bay window with a view of the mountains and Bay Area. There were a lot of side conversations going on between the girls, the hairstylists, and the makeup artist, and the house was vibrating with so much excitement and happiness.

Once our hair and makeup were done, it was time to get dressed. The girls were wearing simple black, sleeveless floor-length dresses with white pearl earrings. They carried a bouquet of white tulips while my bouquet was made of lilies, mixed flowers, and green leaves as a tribute to the flowers Gary had bought me when we first met. Gary helped Pat get his tuxedo tie on, and then the other groomsmen arrived dressed and ready. After taking some photos in our living room, we folded ourselves into the limos and headed off to the ceremony.

When we arrived at the church, Gary opened the door of the limo with a wide swing and came out with a huge smile, his arms raised as he stepped out and waved to everyone. He was beaming with pride and happiness as he shouted, "This is the best day of my life!" I couldn't help but feel the same way.

Soon, it was time to meet my husband-to-be at the altar. My son Pat walked me down the aisle to the song "Here Comes the Bride," and I was overcome with emotion as we passed by our friends and family, who smiled and wished us congratulations.

Finally, I stood next to Gary and the minister at the altar. Gary and I read a poem to each other, the minister gave us his blessings, and then there was a silence. The minister had told us that he might sing after pronouncing us as man and wife, but he couldn't promise since it depended on the strength of his voice that day. To our surprise and delight, the minister sang the song "All I Ask of You" from *The Phantom of the Opera* in an operatic voice. It was the most moving and beautiful rendition I'd heard, and as the tears flowed down my cheeks, I held Gary's hands tight so that I didn't sob in front of everyone.

Gary and I were now married after all these years of commitment, and it was time for the reception. The Roundhill Country Club was a familiar place for us since we had been members for the past seven years, but this time we entered the building as a married couple, ready to celebrate our wedding and Gary's sixtieth birthday. We mixed with our guests during the cocktail party, and for dinner we shared a table with our adult children and their significant others. We were thrilled that so many of our friends and family could join us, including many friends from years past—especially Gary's fraternity brothers.

The band played a mixture of disco and Motown music, and they allowed Gary to sing along at times. As the night went on, there was a large group line dance and even a group wave after one of the songs. It was a lot of fun, and I was especially pleased when Liz caught my bridal bouquet.

One of the highlights of our celebration was when Gary got up on the stage with the band and sang "Pretty Woman" as I danced in front of him with my friends. Everyone stood up with raised arms and swayed back and forth with the music, and then some people joined us on the floor, laughing and dancing. It truly was the best day of our lives.

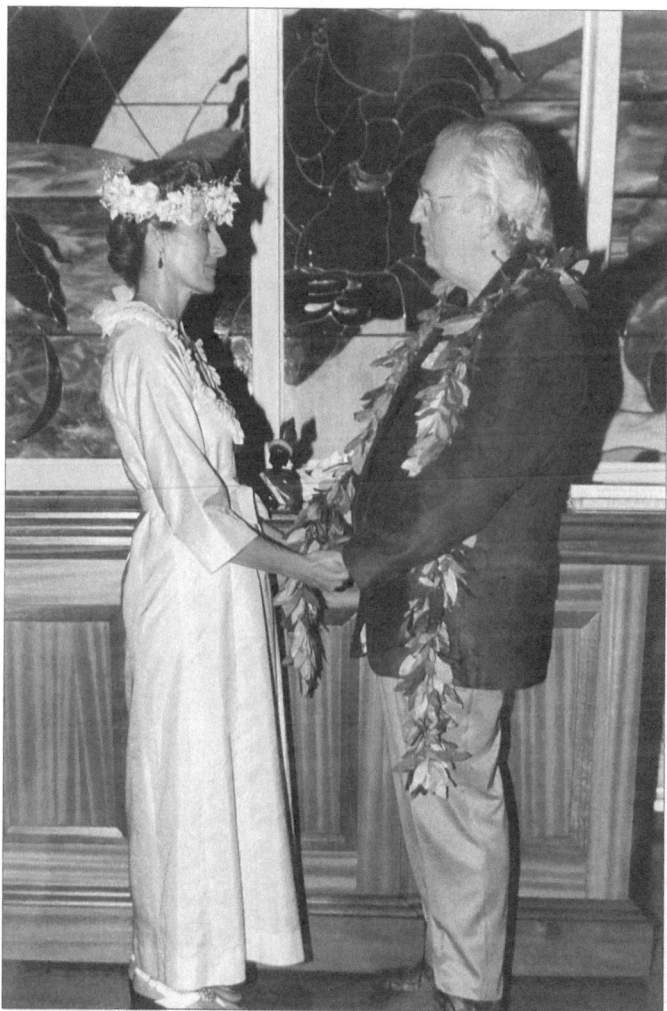

The commitment ceremony, Maui, 1995

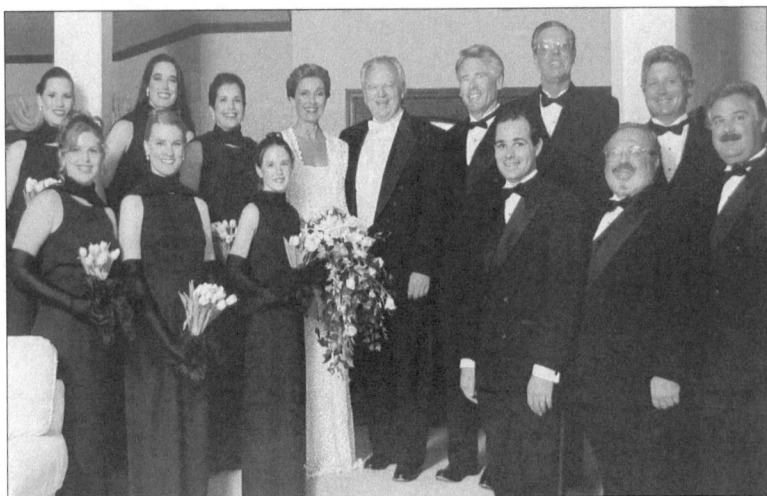

Lilly and Gary's wedding party, 1997
Photo by Greta Heintz, photographer, Walnut Creek, CA

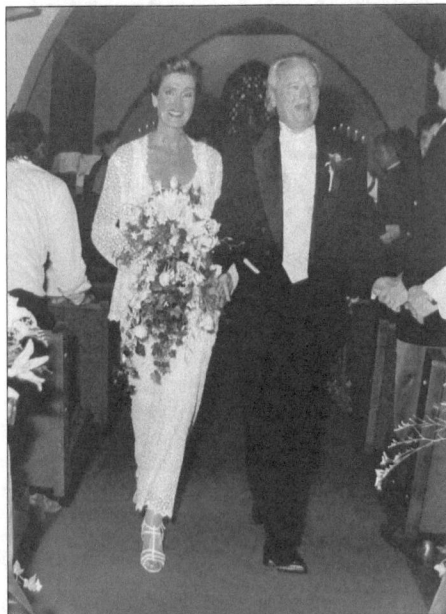

Lilly and Gary's wedding, 1997
Photo by Greta Heintz,
photographer,
Walnut Creek, CA

EIGHTEEN

A Return to Africa

A year after we were married, Gary and I were on our way to Africa for a three-week safari adventure with Liz, Catherine, and Jen so that we could share a place that we loved with them. This was going to be a time for us to get to know our daughters on an even more intimate level. Unfortunately, Pat and Lisa were unable to join us on this trip.

After a long flight, we were met at the airport in Johannesburg, South Africa, by a private car company that then brought us to a home called Waterhouse where we would be staying for two nights. Gary and I had chosen a travel agency that could set us up in the homes of British colonists as we thought this would be the perfect place to relax and recover from our jet lag before going out into the bush. This house was owned by a couple named Ingrid and John, and we were their only guests.

When we entered the suburban home, a maid guided us to our rooms. Gary and I had a separate guest suite while the girls were on the other side of the house, with Liz having her own space and Catherine and Jen sharing a room.

Ingrid was a very pleasant-looking woman in her early fifties with soft blond hair and blue eyes. She welcomed us, then gave us a tour to help us feel at home. She showed us where to find snacks such as ice cream, cookies, chips, soda, and wine, and Gary and I noticed the girls looking at each other with impish eye rolls and smiles. They were conservative young girls from our viewpoint, but the way they were looking at each other made us wonder what they might get up to.

We felt safe and comfortable in our guest house, but a sense of unease came over us when we headed out to a local restaurant for dinner. The house was surrounded by a barbed wire fence with electric devices to keep out intruders. Ingrid shared with us that she had to stay within certain areas of her house to be safe, and she had to be careful what she said in front of her house staff. At this time, there was a fair amount of tension between the British and the Black Africans. Unemployment was high, and the opportunities for Black Africans remained low. Muggings and carjackings were common occurrences, especially in the downtown area, and travelers were routinely warned to exercise caution when traversing the city by any means. This was one of the reasons we had gone through our travel agency to hire private drivers and stay in private homes.

The next morning, after our breakfast, we all went on a tour of Pretoria and then spent the late afternoon relaxing before we enjoyed a home-cooked meal with Ingrid and John. The girls told us they were looking forward to visiting their first camp the next morning, where they would hopefully get to see the big five animals.

The next three nights were going to be spent camping at Chitabe Camp in Botswana, which was highly recommended by our travel agent and was supposed to be a good place to see the animals. To get there, we flew from Maun International Airport on a small, cramped, twin-engine plane with just enough space for the five of us and the pilot. The flight was quite bumpy; Liz and Jen felt nauseous, and Liz later told us that she was so scared she was fighting back tears. Gary and I felt bad that they both had difficulty flying in the small plane, so we tried to give the two of them time to relax when we first arrived at the camp. They recovered quickly, and soon they were both laughing and celebrating being on the ground.

Our hosts were Charles and Linda, an engaged couple in their late thirties, and the girls enjoyed meeting them since they were close in age. The camp was made up of eight luxury tents built on elevated wooden decks under a canopy of indigenous trees, and I was anxious to see what our tent looked like inside. I was pleased to see we had our own twin-bedded room with an indoor bathroom that included a shower. The girls worked out their own sleeping arrangements, and they decided that Jen and Liz would share a tent while Catherine would have one to herself.

We all unpacked and then met up for afternoon tea. We entered a separate thatched dining room and bar, linked by raised walkways, where we all enjoyed a delicious variety of baked goods and sandwiches along with tea, coffee, and hot chocolate. And after we were done, we took the girls on their first safari game drive. Gary and I were excited for them to experience the wilds of Africa, and we hoped they enjoyed it as much as we did.

For the drive, we had our own private, open four-wheel vehicle along with a driver and a scout. We started our drive at about 4 p.m. so we could explore and look for the big five. The scout was our lookout for the leopards; being nocturnal animals, they were hard to find and see. Once he spotted one, the driver would slow down, quiet his engine, and get as close to the animal as possible. As it became dark, the scout had a large flashlight that he could use to spotlight the animal so we could see it with our binoculars.

On one occasion, we were fortunate to observe a leopard lying on the middle of a tree branch, eating his prey. At the base of the tree, a hyena was walking around the tree trunk eating whatever was dropped by the leopard above. What a beautiful lesson on the cycle of nature.

Back at the camp, we enjoyed sitting around under the thatched bar area and listening to Stretch, the camp's food coordinator, give us a preview of our dinner for the evening. He explained each dish with enthusiasm and a level of detail that made us hungry, our mouths watering and ready to eat. While all the food was delightful, the fresh-baked bread with butter each evening was pure heaven.

On our drive the second evening, we saw a family of elephants walking through the tall brown grass, followed by a young baby who was camouflaged by its surroundings. We also saw a few giraffes, their long necks held high, nipping away at the tree leaves. The nighttime drive felt carefree and relaxing, the cool evening breeze softly touching our faces. Gary and I loved listening to our daughters laughing and trying to be the first to spot an animal.

The following morning, we saw a male cheetah and followed him for a few hours. As he attempted to sneak up on a Cape buffalo, he slouched close to the ground and slowly placed one leg forward at a time, his sleek, muscular limbs primed to pounce. It was exciting to watch and feel the tension of the cheetah in his natural world. We did not get to see him succeed, unfortunately; it could take quite a while for this kill to happen.

We also came across a pride of lions lying around. They lazily lifted their heads to see what was going on, and then most snuggled into one another to fall back asleep while some of the younger lions got up and started to play. None of them seemed to be interested in us as we sat and watched them from our vehicle, even though we were only a few feet away. The guide explained, "They will not be threatened by the vehicle as long as we sit quietly and don't make any sudden moves."

Later, we drove past a watering hole frequented by hippos. We saw several giraffes there as well, and it was amusing to see how one giraffe spread her two front legs while bending down to drink the water.

Toward the end of our night drive, Liz said, "Look! There's a leopard walking across our path." We picked up our binoculars and tried to zoom in on him. He was moving at a quick pace, and we noticed that the tip of his tail curled up at the end. As I mentioned before, leopards are hard to find, so I was happy that Liz was able to spot one on her own.

After three days at this incredible camp, we boarded another twin-engine plane to King's Pool Camp, located outside Chobe National Park in Botswana. Both Liz and Jen did much better on this small plane, and they were pleased with themselves for being able to enjoy this flight. The girls were also thrilled to see a few zebras wandering about the grasslands as we drove to our new campsite.

We arrived at the camp to find nine tented rooms with thatched bathrooms, with each room built on a raised teak deck with a view of the King's Pool lagoon. Gary wanted to come to this camp because of his love of hippos—they were prevalent in this area. Our tents were comfortable, and we all had screens on both ends of our tents to get a view of the lagoon frequented by hippos, elephants, crocodiles, lions, baboons, and monkeys. We were warned that the monkeys and baboons had a tendency to get into your tent and steal your stuff, so we had to be sure to zip up our tents each time we left. We loved walking across the expansive raised decks to the lounge and veranda, which overlooked a lovely lagoon with ebony and Jackalberry trees as well as the Linyanti River. It was peaceful and beautiful here. The five of us would end each day at this camp by sitting around the firepit on the veranda, looking out over the lagoon and talking about the highlights of our day.

Gary and I loved watching our adult children being together and enjoying this time not only with each other but with us as well. This trip helped bring the girls closer together, and we were happy that they truly liked each other's company. There was lots of laughter throughout our days and evenings over silly childhood memories as well as prior trips together. And more recently, Liz and Jen loved teasing Catherine about her interest in one of the cute guides from the previous camp.

I also found that spending this time with Liz helped us heal and strengthen our relationship. Each trip we went on helped bring us closer together and make up for the times in Liz's life when I was not there for her in the way she needed me, mostly after my divorce from her father.

I know Gary felt the same way about going on these trips with his children. Gary's relationship with Jen had always been strong since she had lived with Gary until his separation from his wife, Liz, in 1990. The relationship between Catherine and Gary was a more difficult one, though, as they faced more challenges throughout her early childhood years after Gary divorced his first wife, Georgia. After Gary and I met, Catherine became more involved in his life— and in the lives of his other daughters as well as my own children— and this strengthened their relationship as well. This particular trip deepened not only Catherine's love for Gary, but also Jen, whom she did not spend a lot of time with before now, and Liz. It has been a pleasure for Gary and me to see everyone grow together.

Our first day after arriving, we decided not to go on a game drive. It had been very dusty while driving, and Gary's allergies were acting up. Instead, Gary, Catherine, and I took a three-mile walk on the air strip while Liz and Jen relaxed at the camp, and then we all spent the afternoon writing, reading, and relaxing. It felt good to slow down for a day.

This camp was absolutely wonderful, full of wildlife and sights to see. Liz, Jen, and Catherine enjoyed the safari drives as well as our days of just being with each other. On our last evening, we all went on a double-decker boat tour of the Linyanti River, during which we saw baboons, elephants, hippos, and bushbuck. The entire stay was magical, and we were pleased to be so immersed in nature.

However, we did have one unfortunate event at this camp. During one of the morning game drives, we felt some unusual bumps. Our guide stopped the vehicle to check what was going on and discovered we had a flat tire—even worse, we were out in the middle of nowhere with no spare. The driver had to radio another vehicle to bring us a tire and change it. We learned from this trip that we needed to be resilient, and that no matter where we traveled, there were always people ready to help us when needed. All ended well, and we came away from the event with a story to tell.

※○※

Our next adventure began with a four-hour flight on another small plane from King's Pool to Kasane, Botswana. Upon our arrival, we were picked up by a private car service and had a two-hour drive across the border into Zimbabwe and on to The Victoria Falls Hotel for a two-night stay.

The Victoria Falls Hotel is one of the grandest in all of Africa, originally built by the British in 1904 as accommodations for workers on the Cape to Cairo Railway. After staying in camps for the last while, we looked forward to sleeping in a hotel for a change—while the camps had been lovely, there is nothing like sleeping in a grand historic hotel with fine sheets and towels.

As we entered the lobby, we were met with a feeling of old-fashioned charm. Across from the hotel, we could see the magnificent falls and hear the power of the water crashing against the high rock walls, creating a roar of thunder and a wide spray of water. It was a different sort of natural beauty than what we had been experiencing so far.

The next morning, we made the five-mile walk into Zambia to view the falls from the bridge. As we walked across the bridge, we watched river rafts and boats try to maneuver the powerful currents. Luckily, the boats all had experienced guides helping them avoid the rocks while they were being tossed up in the air by the raging waters. There was also the option to go bungee jumping off the bridge. None of us were willing to do this ourselves, but we had fun living vicariously through the brave people taking part in this thrilling experience. We saw them plunge down a steep ravine toward the water below and could hear them shout and scream as they recoiled back up toward the bottom of the bridge. We ended the day with a delicious dinner in the Livingstone Room, an elegant dining room, before getting ready for our next adventure.

Next on our itinerary was Ruckomechi Camp, an exclusive camp located in a remote area on the western side of the Mana Pools National Park in Zimbabwe. Our travel agent, who was especially knowledgeable about African travel destinations, highly recommended visiting this area, so we decided to add it to our trip.

Our travels started with another small plane experience, but this time Jen and Liz told us they were apprehensive because the pilot had complained about the weight of our bags. To our relief, the two-hour flight ended up being smooth.

We arrived at the airport and were met by a van that took us on a one-and-a-half-hour drive along winding roads. Liz said she was feeling ill from motion sickness, and Jen was tired after all the tension from her fear of flying on the small plane. Fires burned along the road, which they told us was a natural part of weeding out the brush, but they still made us nervous.

After the drive we had a one-and-a-half-hour motorboat ride. The scenery on this part of the trip was much nicer, with us being surrounded by green vegetation and water. The temperature was warm, and by now Jen and Liz were feeling better. Despite all this beauty, I couldn't help but think, *How far is this place?* I knew it was supposed to be remote, but it seemed like we had traveled a very long way.

We finally arrived at the camp and found it to be a serene setting with ten luxury grass huts whose open windows overlooked the Zambezi River. A unique feature of this place was that the windows were covered in wire to keep the animals out while letting air in. The bugs could still get in, though, so there were nets over our beds that we could draw closed during the night. We had some anxiety about tsetse flies and mosquitoes, but we relaxed once we found that they were not a problem.

We arrived midafternoon and were able to relax and have afternoon tea before going on our evening game drive. We were fortunate to see a female and male lion playing in the grass on the side of the road, and we stopped the vehicle to watch them for a while. The female became playful and then they began mating—we were definitely getting the full experience out of this trip!

Liz wanted to see the Cape buffalo, and we were lucky enough to find one. They are a large, dark-brown, hoofed mammal with drooping fringed ears and curved horns. They are extremely social and live in large, mixed herds of up to two thousand members. They are known to be dangerous when they are cornered or injured, so we kept our distance.

The next day, after we went on our morning game drive, I came back to find that I had lost one of my diamond earrings, which Gary had bought for me for our commitment ceremony. Gary found the backing of it under the bathroom sink, and I had heard something fall in the bathroom after the morning drive. We did our best to look for it, but the thatched straw floors made it almost impossible to find the tiny earring. When we reported it to the manager, I was told that the day before, the woman who was staying in our hut also lost a diamond earring that she had been given by her boyfriend. What a coincidence! I hoped to find it before leaving the next day, but I instinctively knew that I had to learn to let go. I never did find it, but the loss was a small blip on an otherwise magnificent trip.

The next harrowing experience came when I joined Gary and Catherine on a one-and-a-half-hour canoe trip down the Zambezi River, which was known to be home to hippos. We'd heard stories of hippos overturning canoes, so Liz and Jen wisely decided that they did not want to join us, but I thought it would be okay. We would have guides with us, so how dangerous could it be?

There were two canoes, one for Gary and me with our guide and another for Catherine and her guide. During one part of the trip, we noticed that there were several hippos in the area. We were told to avoid them by giving them space and canoeing on the other side of them—except there were two crocodiles in that direction who did not move from their place. We also had to avoid tree trunks in the water because hitting them could make us capsize! It was very tense and frightening for a while, knowing that we were in a potentially dangerous situation if our canoe tipped over. We got through the experience, and while I am glad I did it, I would not choose to do it again. This remote camp was the last stop on our trip, so at the end of our stay we all made our way back to the States.

Overall, the trip was a great success. Gary and I were delighted to take our daughters on this safari adventure to further their bonding with each other as sisters and with us as a family. I couldn't wait until we could travel together again, and hopefully bring Pat and Lisa with us as well.

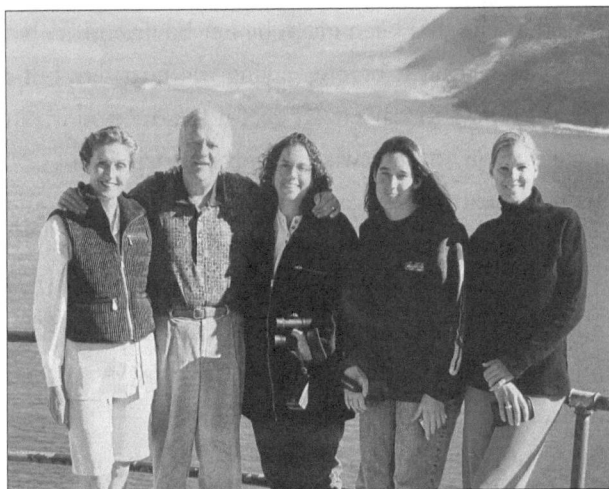

Lilly, Gary, Liz, Jen, and Catherine in Cape Town, 1998

Liz, Jen, Catherine, and Gary in Africa, 1998

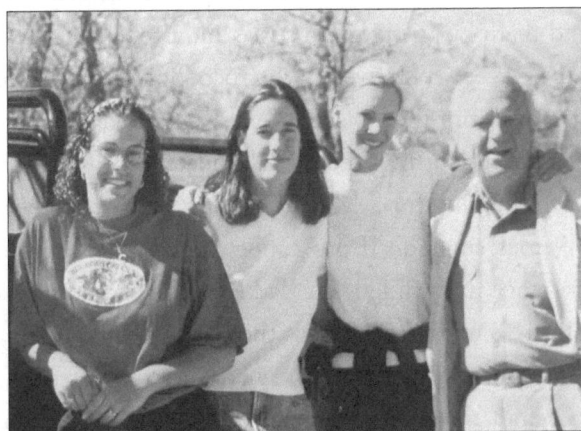

NINETEEN

Becoming Grandparents

E ven though I had a loving and close relationship with my paternal grandparents, especially my grandfather, I had not put much thought into becoming a grandparent myself. Gary did not have a close relationship with his grandparents growing up, so he did not have strong feelings on the matter either. We both felt that having kids was a personal decision that each of our children would make sometime in the future, and we had no bearing on that decision.

Then, in 2002, I got the news that I was going to become a grandmother: Liz and her husband at the time, Todd, were now expecting their first child. I immediately knew exactly how I wanted to be as a grandparent, which was to model myself after my grandfather John: confident, loving, assured, and involved. I was now sixty-one years old, and I felt ready to take on this role. I was working solely as an independent medical legal consultant and was able to have control over my work schedule, so I knew I would be able to make plenty of time for this new addition to our family. Gary was sixty-six and still working full time as a lawyer, so while he was looking forward to being a grandfather, he wouldn't be able to be as involved. He also wasn't quite sure how to be one since he had no role model in his own life.

When I received the call that Liz was on the way to the hospital. I dropped everything and drove to Sacramento to try and be there for the birth. I made it in time to see my granddaughter enter the world, and I was honored to be the one to cut the cord, at Liz's request—Todd was too overwhelmed by it all to do anything but grin. They named her Emily, with the name being a combination of my name and the name of Todd's mother, Mary. I was so proud to watch them slide into their roles as mom and dad. Todd took the role of stay-at-home dad while Liz went back to her position as a social worker about seven weeks later. Todd's mother and father had died a few years earlier, so Gary and I were the primary grandparents for Emily. I was called "Grandma," and Emily named Gary "Pop Pop."

Emily was one of the easiest babies I'd met, a joy from the moment she was born. Even after I'd been a mother and experienced the love that came with it, I had no idea how much I would come to love that little girl. When Emily was a toddler, I would drive up to Sacramento once a week to give Todd a day off and spend time with just the two of us—my favorite thing to do. I'd forgotten how magical the world looked through a child's eyes. With Emily, every shell, every flower, every moment we spent together had a brand-new sparkle to it. I'd take her for a long walk in her stroller and show her the flowers along the way. I'd pick one for her to look at, and we'd gently touch the soft petals. We would look up at the clouds, or she would crawl around in the sand and look at the ladybugs in the bushes. She had a vivid imagination, and I often wondered where her creative interests would take her. Emily also had a gift for art, especially for drawing portraits of family and friends. We still have her earlier drawings hanging up in our home.

Noah, Todd and Liz's second child, came two years later. He was a sweet baby, and my heart expanded even more. As a toddler, Noah was fascinated with bugs, especially lizards and snakes, and he loved going to the zoo.

I continued my weekly time with my grandkids, but Emily had trouble accepting the attention I gave Noah. Whenever I would go to pick Noah up, Emily would run over to me and say "No! No!" while pushing Noah away from my arms. It was hard for her to share this special time we had together, but over time she adjusted to this new reality.

Gary and my third grandchild, Anneke, was born to Catherine and her husband at the time, Cory, in 2005, a year after Noah arrived. She was the first granddaughter on both her mother and father's side of the family, and I loved seeing everyone gather around this small, delicate, beautiful person.

Catherine and her family lived in Houston, so the time we got to spend with Anneke was primarily when we had family get-togethers in the summer or fall. Despite living thousands of miles apart, Anneke and Emily became very close with each other over the ensuing years and talked almost every day as teenagers. Anneke was interested in fashion as a young girl and has a talent for style and makeup as well as writing stories. I look forward to seeing what she pursues as a career.

Benjamin, the first son of Pat and his wife at the time, Jennifer, came a year later in 2006. Ben was Pat's first child but Jennifer's third as she had two children from prior relationships, Zachery and Madison. I spent the day with him once a week like I had done with Emily and Noah, and I soon learned that he was a strong child. He skipped straight over walking to running, and his athletic strength would continue to reveal itself in his pursuit of competitive sports like swimming and football. Pat and Liz lived within walking distance of each other, so I was able to spend a lot of quality time with them and their families.

Ashley came into the family two years after Ben, and as the youngest of four, she was born with the determination to be heard and keep up with her siblings. We loved seeing her excitement in being a cheerleader in grade school as well as when she played volleyball with a traveling team in junior high and as a junior varsity member as a freshman. Even as a young girl, Ashley had an awareness of where everyone in the family was, who they were, where they lived, and their relationships to one another. Ben and Ashley's activities have kept Pat quite busy in addition to his position as a CFO in banking.

Tyler was the fifth grandchild, born shortly after Ben, and the first son for Jen and her husband, Tom. They lived in Virginia and maintained a close relationship with us through family get-togethers and frequent phone conversations. Tyler was a sweet and shy child who showed us from a young age that he was destined to be a strong athlete, especially in lacrosse. His brother Trevor, our seventh grandchild, arrived four years later, and he exhibited his strength in sports from the day he walked. He loves being outdoors, just like his brother and father. You can always find them either skiing, surfboarding, mountain biking, or playing lacrosse or baseball, and Tom does this all while balancing his busy chiropractic practice. Jen has quite the time keeping up with their busy schedules in addition to her own work as a therapist for children at a local grammar school.

Lee, the first son of Lisa and her partner, Ray, is our eighth and last grandchild. Lee was born with a gift for music, and as a toddler he expressed interest in playing the violin. Ray is a musician while Lisa is a creative artist who has worked as a set designer for several years. While she is now studying to be a therapist in mental health, Lee is showing an interest in art as well—he enjoys drawing figures, such as men in battle, and making a story out of them. They lived in New York before settling in Rhode Island, and like Jen, Lisa stays in close touch with her dad and our extended family by joining us on our annual family trips.

The world is wide open to our grandchildren, and as grandparents, Gary and I have enjoyed them at each stage of their development while they explored different activities. We continue to learn about their personalities, how they see the world, and their individual strengths and weaknesses. Each of them will find out where and how they want to be in this world, and we can't wait to see the people they become.

Gary and I have watched our kids grow from children into young adults and now parents. Since they never lived together as young teens or adults, we decided to take them on trips to provide a neutral environment for them to learn more about each other, to great success. Now, fifteen years since our first family vacation, we wanted to continue this tradition with our grandchildren in a place that was mutually acceptable to our adult children.

We decided on having an annual vacation at Pajaro Dunes, California. This was a special place that Gary had enjoyed with his daughters during his marriage to Liz, and all of us loved being here. We rented two large beachfront houses with several bedrooms. Each family had their own separate space yet shared the kitchen, dining room, and living room, and all the families took turns providing dinner. We were close to the ocean, which was especially convenient for those who had to drag along their infant and toddler accessories to camp out on the beach for a few hours.

We started this tradition in 2006 when Zack was eleven, Madison was six, Emily was four, Noah was two, Anneke was one, and Ben was four months. We continued this bonding time together for the next several years, which grew to include Tyler, Ashley, Trevor, and Lee. Despite the boundaries we had set with our own kids in the past—what they could eat, where they could play, when they had to be in bed—Gary and I were able to let each parent discipline their own children. We only had to provide the opportunity for them to be happy and enjoy the fun of everyone being together.

We loved to see Liz and Jen sitting on Liz's infamous red blanket, talking and keeping an eye on the kids as they played along the beach. The red blanket went on every Pajaro Dunes trip, and it ended up being the family meeting point on the beach—it was a great marker for the little ones to look for if and when they roamed away from their parents. Tom would often join them on the blanket, and he and Liz would lightheartedly tease each other. Pat enjoyed sitting on the beach with a book while Ashley played at his side, keeping an eye out for Ben who was known to go off on his own.

Tom loved building sandcastles or surfboarding with the boys. Lisa and Ray would build castles with Lee, along with watching him play with Tyler and Trevor. Catherine would go for runs along the beach while Anneke, Emily, Noah, and Ben were old enough to go up to the house on their own—Ashley, as the youngest, would stay back with her mom or dad. There was always a soft breeze and the sound of seagulls hovering above, with sandpipers running along the beach. The kids would run in and out of the water, chasing each other as waves crashed upon the sand.

We decided to stop going to Pajaro Dunes in 2018 because several of the grandchildren became involved in sports and could not get away for the summer. However, it will always remain a special place in our hearts. It was a place and time where family was important, and where we built love and connection between us. Gary and I loved our time with our family and enjoyed having all the joys of parenthood without the hard work of being a parent.

Our grandchildren remind us how incredible life can be. We're always looking forward to having new adventures and gatherings whenever we can—and as always, we love to find special places to share together.

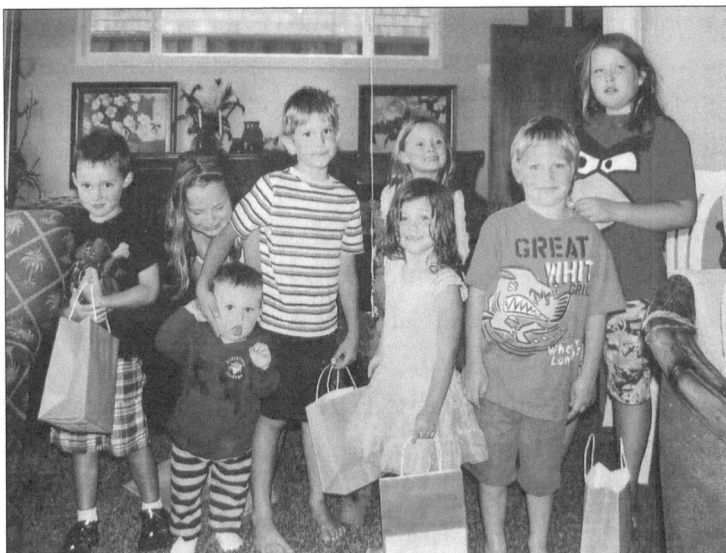

Gary and Lilly's grandchildren at Pajaro Dunes, 2011

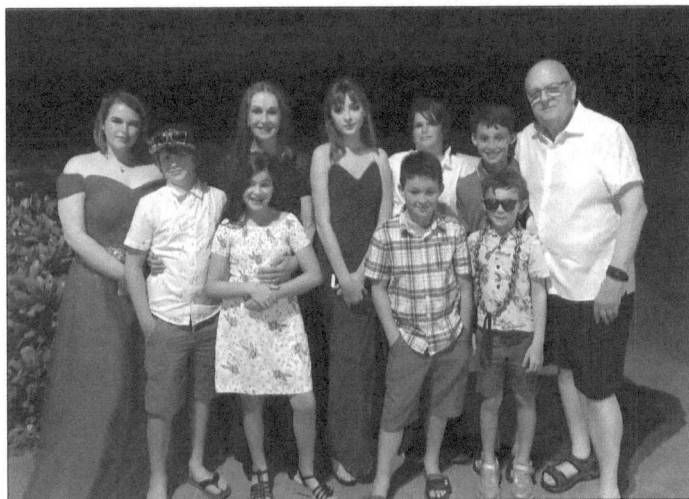

Gary and Lilly with their grandkids in Maui, 2018

Becoming Grandparents

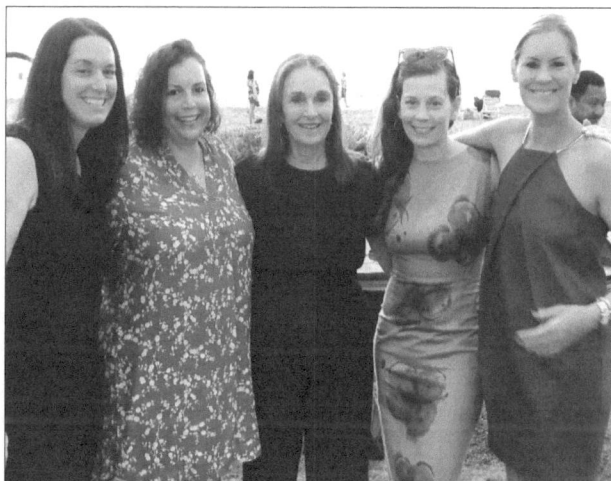

Jen, Liz, Lilly, Lisa, and Catherine in Maui, 2018

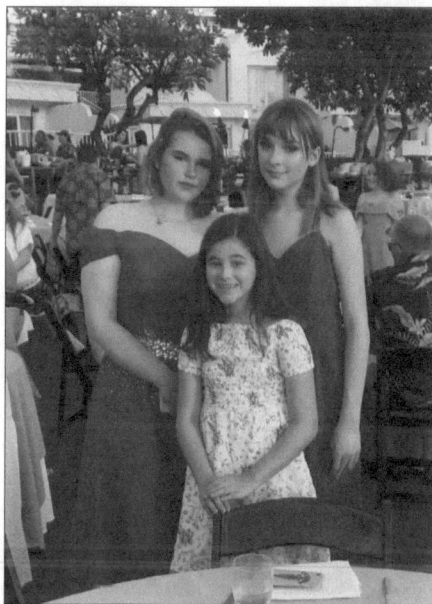

Emily, Anneke, and Ashley in Maui, 2018

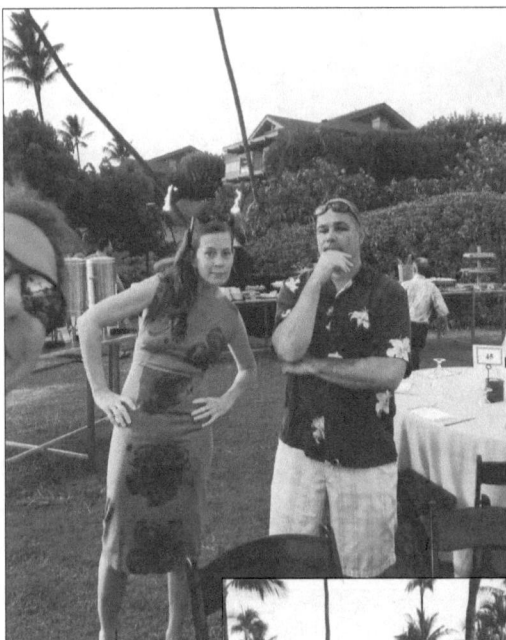

*Lisa, Pat, and Tom
having fun, 2018*

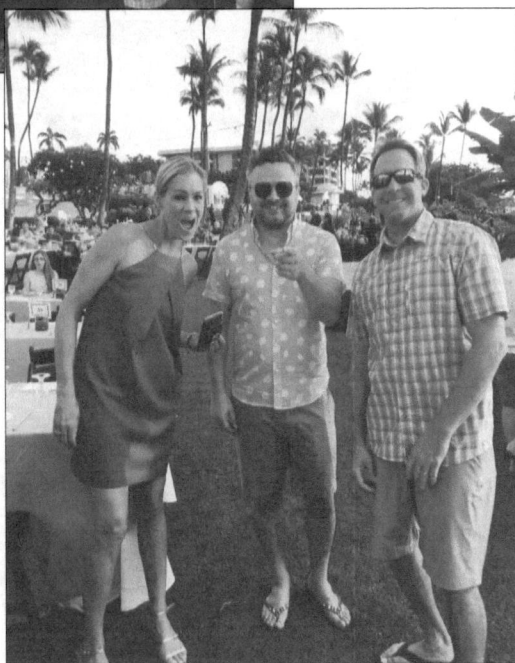

*Catherine, Ray,
and Tom having
fun, 2018*

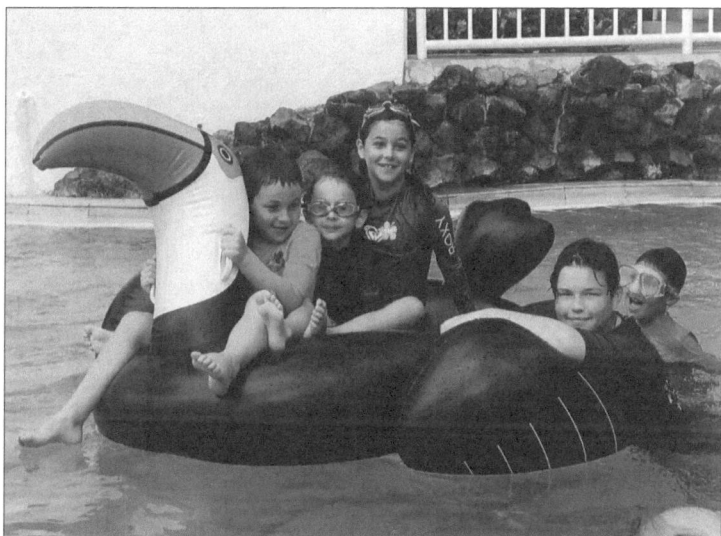

The grandkids having fun in Maui, 2016

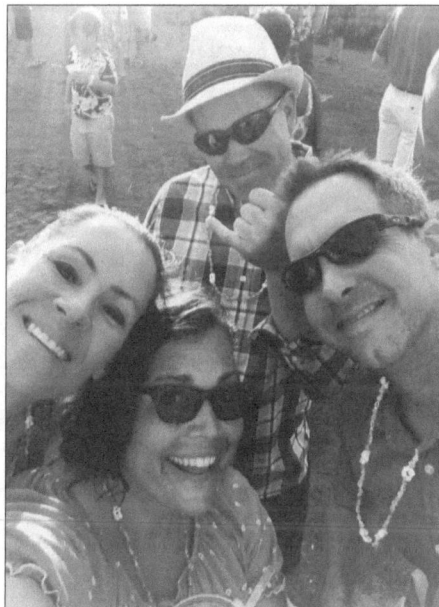

Liz, Catherine, Pat, and Tom in Maui, 2016

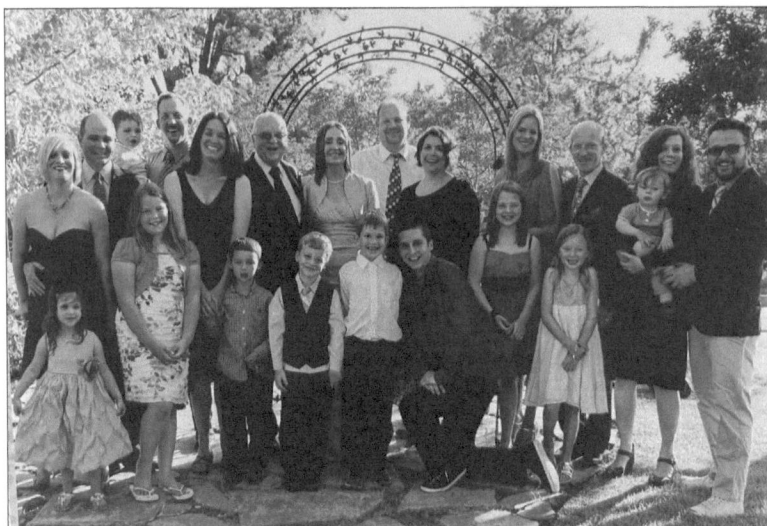

Gary's 75th birthday, 2012

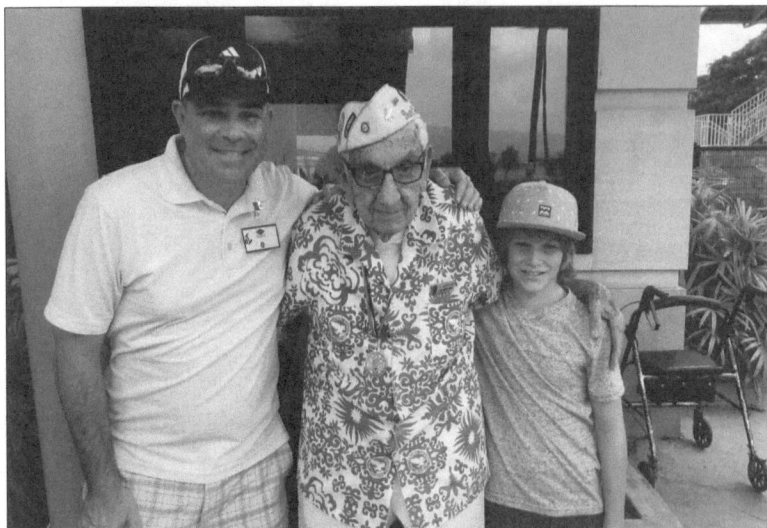

Pat and Ben at Pearl Harbor National Memorial with a veteran, 2016

TWENTY

Coming Full Circle

Our last family trip to Maui was in November 2018, and even now, several years later, our children and grandchildren still talk about their time together in this paradise. We stayed at the Fairmont Kea Lani for two weeks, and each of our five families—seventeen people in total—had an ocean-view room, all on the same floor. The grandchildren ranged in age from seven to sixteen and had a lot more independence to explore the exotic tropical hotel grounds on their own without a parent hovering nearby. What a thrill it was for me to watch all eight grandchildren come and go from one room to another, playing together and huddling in the hall corridors as they decided where they would go next. I always wondered what they were up to and hoped they didn't get into too much mischief.

Their parents were delighted to have the freedom to sit together at the poolside by reserving cabanas and lounge chairs for the day. Liz and Jen became the family leaders, making sure their favorite spots were reserved each morning.

Each day, the morning started with a delicious buffet breakfast. The café overlooked the ocean and pools, and the warm tropical breeze was refreshing. There was a great selection of food to pick from, and Gary and I thoroughly enjoyed seeing our family sitting together and chatting about the day's activities.

As I watched my children handle their own children, I found myself reflecting on my own parenting. I'd been far from a perfect mother; I hadn't always been there for Pat and Liz after divorcing their father, especially when I was obtaining my nursing and law degrees. I'd hoped to make up for this by being fully present as a grandmother, and by sharing these special memories together with all our children. Pat and Liz have often commented on how much more I was available for my grandchildren, and I am thankful that they both allowed me to be such a large part of their kids' lives.

My relationship with Gary's daughters and their spouses was very different. We all live thousands of miles from each other, and of course I'm their stepmother so there is a different dynamic between us. My role as Gary's wife was to support him along with his children and family. Because of that, I felt I needed to establish my own relationship with them, along with their spouses and children, so that they could guide me toward the role they wanted me to play in their lives. I gave permission for their children to call me by any name that was comfortable for them, and I respected that Gary's children might feel differently about my role as a grandmother. I hope I've been able to convey how glad I am that they all came into my life.

Gary has enjoyed his own relationship with each of his daughters, their spouses, and his grandchildren. Over the years, he developed a special relationship with my son and daughter, their spouses, and his grandchildren as well. We see our two families as being combined and each other's children as our own.

Relationships are complicated, and it's difficult to watch people you love struggle in their marriages. Over the years each of our children have faced their own troubles, and in the middle of such heartbreaks we have all worked to make the grandkids feel safe and loved. That's the family foundation that Gary and I started to build when we met in 1990.

Today, as I am writing this book, I think back on Gary and my history together. It was during our first trip to Maui in 1991 that Gary asked me to move to Oakland with him—that was the start of our life together. We've come so far since then, gone so many places, and with each new family event, we've created new memories and new traditions. We continue building our family and finding comfort in each other, and I feel a deeper love grow within our family as each year passes.

As I write this, I am eighty years old, Gary is eighty-five, and we're celebrating our twenty-fifth wedding anniversary this year. There is so much joy to share and so many ways to love in our family. We have come almost full circle with our life journey, and we have written in our will that when the time comes, we want our family to come together once again to scatter our ashes by the ocean at Wailea Point. We can think of no better way to celebrate our time together—to be with our family once more in the place it all began.

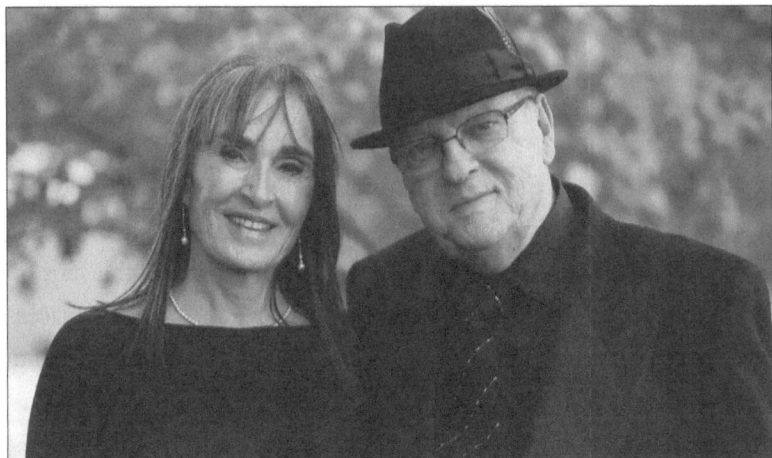

Lilly and Gary, celebrating 75th and 80th birthdays, 2017
Photo by Chris Sentovich, photographer, San Jose, CA

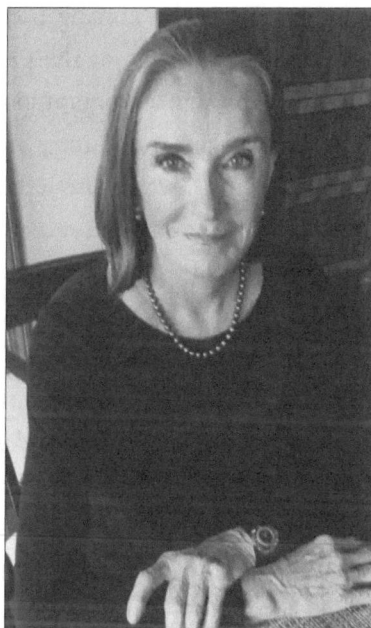

ABOUT THE AUTHOR

Lilly A. Gwilliam has held a variety of positions over the course of her life, including working as a medical legal consultant, a dean of allied health, an accreditation officer, a nursing coordinator, a practitioner teacher, and a psychiatric nurse. She is also a speaker, having presented a paper on rape to the Fiji Law Society, and was able to help change the laws around rape in Fiji. Additionally, she presented a seminar on the elimination of gender bias in the legal profession at the University of Cape Town Law School in Africa and at several law conferences in California.

Lilly has been inducted into the nursing honor society Sigma Theta Tau. She was nominated as one of the Outstanding Young Women of America in 1979 through a program sponsored by leading women's organizations throughout the country and is a member in *Who's Who in American Nursing*. Lilly was also inducted into the 2014 Massapequa High School Hall of Fame in recognition of her commitment to excellence in her profession as she honors her responsibilities to her family and community.

As a writer, Lilly authored the memoir *Generations of Motherhood: A Changing Story* and has published a chapter in the book *Women of Worth: Emotional Intelligence – Mental Health Matters* by Christine Awram. She has also published several articles on the topics of nursing and law.

Lilly currently lives in Alamo, California, with her husband, Gary. They have five children and eight grandchildren between them, and they enjoy spending time with their family and traveling the world.

Website: www.lillygwilliam.com

Email: lilly@lillygwilliam.com

LinkedIn: www.linkedin.com/in/lilly-gwilliam-0ba21336

Facebook: www.facebook.com/lagwilliam

Instagram: www.instagram.com/lillygwilliam

Made in United States
Troutdale, OR
05/05/2025

31096267R00116